Women's Mental Health:
A Framework for Its Assessment, Prevention, and Promotion in Health Care Settings

Women's Mental Health: A Framework for Its Assessment, Prevention, and Promotion in Health Care Settings

Editors

Carmela Mento
Maria Catena Silvestri

MDPI • Basel • Beijing • Wuhan • Barcelona • Belgrade • Manchester • Tokyo • Cluj • Tianjin

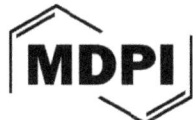

Editors
Carmela Mento
University of Messina
Italy

Maria Catena Silvestri
University of Messina
Italy

Editorial Office
MDPI
St. Alban-Anlage 66
4052 Basel, Switzerland

This is a reprint of articles from the Special Issue published online in the open access journal *International Journal of Environmental Research and Public Health* (ISSN 1660-4601) (available at: https://www.mdpi.com/journal/ijerph/special_issues/Women_Mental).

For citation purposes, cite each article independently as indicated on the article page online and as indicated below:

LastName, A.A.; LastName, B.B.; LastName, C.C. Article Title. *Journal Name* **Year**, *Volume Number*, Page Range.

ISBN 978-3-0365-4119-8 (Hbk)
ISBN 978-3-0365-4120-4 (PDF)

© 2022 by the authors. Articles in this book are Open Access and distributed under the Creative Commons Attribution (CC BY) license, which allows users to download, copy and build upon published articles, as long as the author and publisher are properly credited, which ensures maximum dissemination and a wider impact of our publications.

The book as a whole is distributed by MDPI under the terms and conditions of the Creative Commons license CC BY-NC-ND.

Contents

About the Editors vii

Preface to "Women's Mental Health: A Framework for Its Assessment, Prevention, and Promotion in Health Care Settings" ix

Clemente Cedro, Carmela Mento, Maria Cristina Piccolo, Fiammetta Iannuzzo, Amelia Rizzo, Maria Rosaria Anna Muscatello and Gianluca Pandolfo
Sexual Desire and Body Image. Gender Differences and Correlations before and during COVID-19 Lockdown
Reprinted from: *Int. J. Environ. Res. Public Health* **2022**, *19*, 4351, doi:10.3390/ijerph19074351 . . 1

Alice Mannocci, Sara Ciavardini, Federica Mattioli, Azzurra Massimi, Valeria D'Egidio, Lorenza Lia, Franca Scaglietta, Andrea Giannini, Roberta Antico, Barbara Dorelli, Alessandro Svelato, Luigi Orfeo, Pierluigi Benedetti Panici, Antonio Ragusa, Giuseppe La Torre and HAPPY MAMA Group
HAPPY MAMA Project (Part 2)—Maternal Distress and Self-Efficacy: A Pilot Randomized Controlled Field Trial
Reprinted from: *Int. J. Environ. Res. Public Health* **2022**, *19*, 1461, doi:10.3390/ijerph19031461 . . . 13

Giulia Lausi, Benedetta Barchielli, Jessica Burrai, Anna Maria Giannini and Clarissa Cricenti
Italian Validation of the Scale of Psychological Abuse in Intimate Partner Violence (EAPA-P)
Reprinted from: *Int. J. Environ. Res. Public Health* **2021**, *18*, 12717, doi:10.3390/ijerph182312717 . 29

Maria Di Blasi, Gaia Albano, Giulia Bassi, Elisa Mancinelli, Cecilia Giordano, Claudia Mazzeschi, Chiara Pazzagli, Silvia Salcuni, Gianluca Lo Coco, Omar Carlo Gioacchino Gelo, Gloria Lagetto, Maria Francesca Freda, Giovanna Esposito, Barbara Caci, Aluette Merenda and Laura Salerno
Factors Related to Women's Psychological Distress during the COVID-19 Pandemic: Evidence from a Two-Wave Longitudinal Study
Reprinted from: *Int. J. Environ. Res. Public Health* **2021**, *18*, 11656, doi:10.3390/ijerph182111656 . 43

Jiyoung Song and Eunwon Lee
Health-Related Quality of Life of Elderly Women with Fall Experiences
Reprinted from: *Int. J. Environ. Res. Public Health* **2021**, *18*, 7804, doi:10.3390/ijerph18157804 . . 55

Alice Mannocci, Azzurra Massimi, Franca Scaglietta, Sara Ciavardini, Michela Scollo, Claudia Scaglione and Giuseppe La Torre
HAPPY MAMA Project (PART 1). Assessing the Reliability of the Italian Karitane Parenting Confidence Scale (KPCS-IT) and Parental Stress Scale (PSS-IT): A Cross-Sectional Study among Mothers Who Gave Birth in the Last 12 Months
Reprinted from: *Int. J. Environ. Res. Public Health* **2021**, *18*, 4066, doi:10.3390/ijerph18084066 . . . 65

María Crespo, María Arinero and Carmen Soberón
Analysis of Effectiveness of Individual and Group Trauma-Focused Interventions for Female Victims of Intimate Partner Violence
Reprinted from: *Int. J. Environ. Res. Public Health* **2021**, *18*, 1952, doi:10.3390/ijerph18041952 . . 77

Marcello Passarelli, Laura Casetta, Luca Rizzi and Raffaella Perrella
Responses to Stress: Investigating the Role of Gender, Social Relationships, and Touch Avoidance in Italy
Reprinted from: *Int. J. Environ. Res. Public Health* **2021**, *18*, 600, doi:10.3390/ijerph18020600 . . . 95

Carmenrita Infortuna, Francesco Gratteri, Andrew Benotakeia, Sapan Patel, Alex Fleischman, Maria Rosaria Anna Muscatello, Antonio Bruno, Rocco Antonio Zoccali, Eileen Chusid, Zhiyong Han and Fortunato Battaglia
Exploring the Gender Difference and Predictors of Perceived Stress among Students Enrolled in Different Medical Programs: A Cross-Sectional Study
Reprinted from: *Int. J. Environ. Res. Public Health* **2020**, *17*, 6647, doi:10.3390/ijerph17186647 . . . **109**

Carmela Mento, Maria Catena Silvestri, Maria Rosaria Anna Muscatello, Amelia Rizzo, Laura Celebre, Martina Praticò, Rocco Antonio Zoccali and Antonio Bruno
Psychological Impact of Pro-Anorexia and Pro-Eating Disorder Websites on Adolescent Females: A Systematic Review
Reprinted from: *Int. J. Environ. Res. Public Health* **2021**, *18*, 2186, doi:10.3390/ijerph18042186 . . . **117**

About the Editors

Carmela Mento

Carmela Mento, Prof, a psychologist and Jungian psychoanalyst, has a Ph.D. in psychiatric science. She is an associate professor of clinical psychology, and currently works at the Department of Biomedical and Dental Sciences and Morphofunctional Imaging at the University of Messina, Italy. She is also a clinical psychologist, consultant and supervisor at the Psychiatric Unit at the Policlinico University Hospital, Messina, Italy. Her scientific publishing is centered on psychological diagnosis and psychopathology, assessment and consulting in a medical setting and healthcare, women's mental health, suicide risk, personality disorders, eating disorders, adolescent mental health, and aggressive and violent behavior in healthcare.

Maria Catena Silvestri

Maria Catena Silvestri, Psy.D., is a Ph.D. student at the University of Messina, Italy. She is a psychotherapist, and her scientific interests have focused on developmental psychopathology, child and adolescent mental health and psychotherapy treatments, developmental disorders and autism, and psychological and psychiatric rehabilitation.

Preface to "Women's Mental Health: A Framework for Its Assessment, Prevention, and Promotion in Health Care Settings"

The psychological assessment and prevention of women's mental health brings attention to the female condition, which is currently affected by greater attention being devoted to the quality of couples' lives as well as important social educational aspects in the prevention and recognition of psychological and physical violence. Wellbeing promotion in healthcare settings is needed to increase knowledge and promote positive attitudes towards women's mental health, also in relation to the promotion of training and assistance courses based on gender medicine.

Carmela Mento and Maria Catena Silvestri
Editors

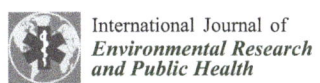

Article

Sexual Desire and Body Image. Gender Differences and Correlations before and during COVID-19 Lockdown

Clemente Cedro [1], Carmela Mento [1], Maria Cristina Piccolo [2], Fiammetta Iannuzzo [1], Amelia Rizzo [3,*], Maria Rosaria Anna Muscatello [1] and Gianluca Pandolfo [1]

[1] Department of Biomedical, Dental and Morphological and Functional Imaging Sciences, University Hospital "G. Martino", 98124 Messina, Italy; clemente.cedro@unime.it (C.C.); cmento@unime.it (C.M.); f.iannuzzo@libero.it (F.I.); maria.muscatello@unime.it (M.R.A.M.); gianluca.pandolfo@unime.it (G.P.)
[2] Provincial Health Agency 5, 98123 Messina, Italy; cristina-piccolo@libero.it
[3] Psychiatry Unit, University Hospital "G. Martino", 98124 Messina, Italy
* Correspondence: amrizzo@unime.it

Citation: Cedro, C.; Mento, C.; Piccolo, M.C.; Iannuzzo, F.; Rizzo, A.; Muscatello, M.R.A.; Pandolfo, G. Sexual Desire and Body Image. Gender Differences and Correlations before and during COVID-19 Lockdown. *Int. J. Environ. Res. Public Health* **2022**, *19*, 4351. https://doi.org/10.3390/ijerph19074351

Academic Editor: Cheng-Fang Yen

Received: 28 February 2022
Accepted: 24 March 2022
Published: 5 April 2022

Publisher's Note: MDPI stays neutral with regard to jurisdictional claims in published maps and institutional affiliations.

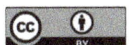

Copyright: © 2022 by the authors. Licensee MDPI, Basel, Switzerland. This article is an open access article distributed under the terms and conditions of the Creative Commons Attribution (CC BY) license (https://creativecommons.org/licenses/by/4.0/).

Abstract: Recent literature has extensively examined sexual behavior during lockdown due to COVID-19. However, there are no recent studies that have considered the relationship between body image quality, sexual arousability, and sexual anxiety. The present study has two main objectives: (1) to examine gender differences in bodily and sexual experience; and (2) the comparison of bodily and sexual experience, before and during the COVID-19 lockdown. A total of 301 adult subjects (161 women and 140 men) aged between 16 and 73 years (Mean = 37.4; S.D. = 10.3) participated in the study. Data on biographical information were collected via an online panel. The Body Uneasiness Test (BUT) and the Sexual Arousability Inventory (SAI) were used for the assessment. Univariate ANOVA showed worse scores for women, compared with men, in terms of body image avoidance, depersonalization, overall severity of body image quality, sexual arousability, and sexual anxiety dimensions. When compared against time, only women showed significant correlations between the function of sexual arousal and all parameters concerning body image alteration. Interestingly, these correlations were weak and sporadic before lockdown, but strong and numerous during lockdown. This finding suggests that the impact of COVID-19 restrictions affected the female population more, with a profound repercussion on self-image and sexual and mental well-being.

Keywords: women; COVID-19; sexuality; body image

1. Introduction

The COVID-19 pandemic has affected people's sex lives. The lockdown period has radically changed interpersonal and inter-partner habits. Many factors such as the fear of contagion, the reduction of social relationships, higher chance of interpersonal conflicts, stress, lack of privacy, and the continued presence of children at home, have impacted sexual quality of life [1]. This has been evidenced by several multinational empirical data on the impact of restrictions and physical distancing on the quality of intimate life, although the nature of those changes does not appear homogeneous, and the issue is still unclear.

During this period of widespread movement and social contact restrictions, on average, the frequency of sexual behavior decreased. A recent study by Lehmiller et al. [2], on a English speaking sample mostly from the United States, 69% of whom were living with a partner and 31% were living alone, showed that many participants (43.5%) reported a decrease in sexual life quality; however, 42.8% reported that it remained the same, or even improved (13.6%). In particular, one in five participants reported expanding their sexual repertoire by incorporating new activities. Common additions included sexting, trying new sexual positions, and sharing sexual fantasies. Participants who made new additions were three times more likely to report improvements in their sex lives. Even in the face of drastic changes to daily life, many adults adapted their sex lives in more creative ways.

Coombe et al. [3] also showed different sexual behaviors during lockdown in the Australian population. More specifically, authors found that most of the participants (53.5%) reported less sex during lockdown, compared with 2019. Thirty-five percent of participants were more likely to report sex with their spouse, and 45% were less likely to report sex with their partners or casual sex.

Another study highlighted the decline in sexual arousal, specifically assessing the impact of COVID-19 measures on partner relationships and reproductive health in China. A sample of 3500 Chinese youth was recruited and interviewed about sexual desire, frequency of sexual intercourse, sexual satisfaction, etc. The questionnaire also collected demographic data (e.g., age, ethnicity, education, current financial situation, sexual orientation, relationship status, etc.). Due to the COVID-19 pandemic and related containment measures, 22% of participants (n = 212) reported a decrease in sexual desire; 41% (n = 396) reported a decrease in the frequency of sexual intercourse; 30% (n = 291) reported an increase in the frequency of masturbation; 20% (n = 192) reported a decrease in alcohol consumption before or during sexual activities; and 31% (n = 298) reported a deterioration in their relationship with their partner during the pandemic. These results show that many Chinese youths experienced significant changes during the lockdown, which affected their sexual and reproductive health [4].

Another study conducted in the United Kingdom examined a sample of 868 individuals during social self-isolation due to COVID-19, in which 39.9% of the sample reported engaging in at least one sexual activity once a week. Being male, a younger age, married, using alcohol frequently, and a greater number of days in self-isolation were associated with greater sexual activity, compared with women. Notably, 60.1% of the sample studied reported not being sexually active during social self-isolation [5].

The heterogeneity of results on sexual behavior during quarantine lead to the hypothesis that other psychological factors can mediate sexual well-being, satisfaction, and relationship quality, such as body image quality. Nevertheless, these studies reported sexual behavior alterations without considering one's relationship with body image. Indeed, it is well known that interpersonal and sexual relationships are influenced by the relationship with the self and body [6,7]. Thus, it can be hypothesized that changes in sexual behavior during the lockdown may be tied to body image alteration, but this interesting hypothesis is still largely unexplored and deserves further analysis.

Body image has been defined as "the personal mental image of the shape, size and dimension of the body and the feelings we have about these characteristics and individual physical parts" [8,9]. Although it is experienced in the third person, body image cannot reach full objectivity, as it is influenced by personal attitudes, and various affective and behavioral components that ultimately modify the individual experience, thus impacting the self-esteem of the subject in particular [10]. Thus, it is the appraisals and emotions related to the experience of one's body that ultimately determine an individual's body satisfaction [11,12]. In the clinical setting, poor body satisfaction is linked to the onset and maintenance of eating or dysmorphic disorders [13], depression [14], anxiety [15], and substance use [16]. It has also been found in several independent studies that women generally report significantly lower levels of body satisfaction [17–19], resulting in a greater vulnerability to these issues.

The body image of each individual plays a key role in the sexual experience because it decisively contributes to sexual confidence. The possibility of feeling, or not feeling, satisfied with one's own body determines a series of behaviors that inevitably reflect on sexuality [20]. The body is the vehicle of sexuality, it is mainly expressed with the body. A negative body image leads to low self-esteem, low body esteem, and dissatisfaction in one's relationship with self-image and others [21]. Literature shows specific gender differences: on the one hand, women are more concerned about weight and body shape; on the other hand, men, in general, tend to be much more focused on the size of the genitals [22].

Scientific evidence suggests that there are gender differences in the perception of body image, in particular, greater body dissatisfaction and greater concerns about body shape have been found in women, rather than in men [23]. In addition, Dang et al. [24] found that sexual anxiety is mediated by factors such as sexual beliefs and attachment, and that this creates complex patterns, which take on different configurations in women and men.

The impact of the coronavirus has been undoubtedly crucial for people's sex lives. It can be hypothesized that its effects will persist in the coming months or years, leading to unpredictable changes in relationships at all levels, not only in terms of affectivity but also in terms of sexual relationships. Psychological, social, and biological factors should be studied, especially regarding the possible increase in sexual desire disorders related to fear or anxiety. The possible reflections on the effects of lockdown in the relational and emotional sphere are indeed numerous, but unfortunately, there are still no systematic studies that have considered sexual behavior concerning body image quality during the pandemic.

Given these premises, the overall purpose of the present study is to investigate the possible effects of lockdown from COVID-19 on body experience, and the possible implications related to sexual functioning in the components of sexual desire, arousal, and anxiety. The specific objectives are (H1) to compare experiences before and during lockdown, taking into account the gender variable; and (H2) to verify the correlations between the different variables before and during, in the female sample.

2. Method

2.1. Procedure

The participants were invited to participate in the survey through mailing lists, instant messaging apps, and posts on Facebook groups, on a voluntary basis. Data were collected between June and October 2020 through Google's telematics platform Forms ©. The research guaranteed anonymity, as requested by the ethical principles stated in the Declaration of Helsinki regarding subjects involved in research. The present survey did not involve any manipulation or treatment of data.

Each participant, before completion, read and signed the informed consent form, in which the purpose of the research was explained: "The School of Psychiatry of Messina University (Italy), is investigating sexual excitability and anxiety associated with body image in relation to the lockdown period for COVID-19 Pandemic. We are interested in how body image-related discomfort, avoidant behaviors and compulsive control may affect people's sexual life. You will be asked to answer short questionnaires. The survey will take about 15 min and respect anonymity and personal information, according to the current privacy law. The collected data will be used only for scientific research purposes. If you are under 18 years, you must ask your parents for consent. If you are taking the survey via cell phone, you will need to put your screen horizontally to view all response options. Thanks for your cooperation".

Subsequently, the subjects were asked to fill out the biographical form containing general information on educational qualifications, occupation and marital status, as well as on romantic relationships and the two rating scales, in a single session lasting 15–30 min. The participants were asked to fill in the questionnaire, thinking retrospectively about their sexual and bodily experiences before the COVID-19 pandemic, and were then asked to give a score that compared them with the same experiences *during* the lockdown. The raw data were entered into an Excel spreadsheet for scoring, and were recoded and processed with the SPSS 25.0 Statistical Package for the Social Sciences (IBM-SPSS Inc., Chicago, IL, USA).

2.2. Instruments

The following two psychodiagnostic instruments were used to assess the variables considered. The Body Uneasiness Test (BUT) [25] is an assessment scale used for the study of body image and its pathologies. It is composed of 34 clinical items and 37 items related to specific experiences of body parts that consider the following dimensions: dissatisfaction and concern about one's weight; concerns with body image; avoidance behaviors; compulsive control behaviors; feelings of detachment and estrangement from the body. Items are rated on a 6-point scale, from 0 (never) to 5 (always); higher scores indicate greater impairment. Several scores, indices, and factors can be obtained. Factor analysis isolated 5 factors (see Figure 1):

Weight Phobia (WP-Weight Phobia)	the sum of scores for items 9, 10, 18, 21, 24, 31, 32, and 33 divided by 8.
Body Image Concerns (BIC)	the sum of item scores 3, 4, 6, 12, 15, 22, 23, 25, and 34 divided by 9.
Avoidance Behavior (A-Avoidance)	the sum of the score of items 5, 8, 13, 16, 19, and 30 divided by 6.
Compulsive Self-Monitoring (CSM-Compulsive Self-Monitoring)	the sum of the score of items 1, 2, 11, 17, 20 and 27 divided by 6.
Depersonalization (D-Depersonalization)	the sum of the score of items 7, 14, 26, 28 and 29 divided by 5.

Figure 1. BUT factors.

In addition to the total score, the Global Severity Index (GSI), or overall mean score, is calculated by summing the clinical scale scores and dividing by their number (34).

The second psychodiagnostic instrument used was the Sexual Arousability Inventory (SAI) [26]. This scale was created to assess the extent of arousal from different sexual experiences. The same instrument, in the so-called "expanded" version (Sexual Arousability Inventory-Expanded-SAI-E) used by us, can assess both the sexual arousability and anxiety that is aroused by the same sexual experiences. The scale, a self-assessment, is composed of 28 items that propose a series of situations of sexual involvement, in which the subject must say to what extent they are made excited or anxious. Each item is rated on a 7-point scale, from −1 (inhibition of arousal or relaxing effect) to 5 (constantly and extremely arousing, or constantly and extremely anxiety-provoking). The total score is obtained by summing the individual item scores (and subtracting the −1 scores). The higher the score, the greater the excitability or anxiety. In the present study, the SAI scale was replicated to provide four experimental conditions: (1) excitability before COVID-19; (2) sexual anxiety before COVID-19; (3) excitability during quarantine; and (4) sexual anxiety during quarantine.

2.3. Participants

The interview was completed by a total of 301 participants, including 140 males and 161 females, ranging in age from 16 to 73 years (mean 37.4; S.D. 10.3); 2.6% (n = 8) of the participants stated that they suffered from a psychiatric pathology; 14.2% (n = 43) of the participants stated that they had undergone cosmetic surgery.

The sociodemographic variables examined are shown in Table 1.

Table 1. Sociodemographic characteristics of the sample.

Sentimental Status	No relationship	11%
	In a stable relationship	66.4%
	In a complicated relationship	9.6%
	In an open relationship	4.7%
	Occasional relationship	8.3%
Profession	Student	8.3%
	Employee	44.9%
	Self-employed	35.5%
	Unemployed	5.6%
	Other	5.6%
Education	Primary school certificate	3.1%
	Secondary school certificate	6.9%
	High School Diploma	25.9%
	Degree	64.1%
Income range	From EUR 0 to 36.152	57.5%
	From EUR 36.153 to 70.000	29.6%
	From EUR 70.001 to 100.000	10.2%
	Over EUR 100.000	2.7%

3. Results

3.1. Statistical Analysis

Statistical analysis was performed using SPSS software version 25.0 for Windows. Descriptive statistics included a calculation of mean values (±SD) for all variables considered. Univariate ANOVA was used to assess changes in scores within the same sample before and during the lockdown. Spearman's test was used for correlation analysis. After Bonferroni correction, p values less than 0.05 were considered statistically significant.

3.2. Gender Differences

The first objective of the study was (H1) to compare the experience before and during the lockdown, taking into account the gender variable. The ANOVA test showed the significant impact of gender on body image and sexual related variables. Therefore, the groups of women and men were analyzed separately, with different results.

In the female group, both body variables, sexual arousal, and anxiety were significantly worse when comparing before and during the lockdown, with statistically significant differences. More specifically, a difference emerged in the following areas of bodily experience: avoidance behavior, depersonalization, and global severity index. On the other hand, weight phobia and compulsive self-image control are at the limits of significance ($p = 0.05$). Moreover, concerning sexual experience, there was a reduction in desire and an increase in anxiety (see Table 2).

Table 2. Comparison of body variables and sexual arousal and anxiety before and during the lockdown in Women.

Women's Scores ($n = 161$)		Mean	Std. Deviation	F	Sig
Weight Phobia	before	1.9	1.2	3.661	0.057
	during	2.2	1.7		
Body Image Concern	before	1.7	1.2	1.668	0.197
	during	1.9	1.6		
Avoidance	before	8.7	1.0	4.885	0.028
	during	1.2	1.6		
Compulsive self-monitoring	before	1.4	1.0	3.669	0.056
	during	1.7	1.5		
Depersonalization	before	0.8	1.1	5.702	0.018
	during	1.2	1.7		
Global Severity Index	before	1.4	1.0	3.937	0.048
	during	1.7	1.5		
Sexual Arousability	before	113.24	32.43	13.984	0.000
	during	97.50	42.43		
Sexual Anxiety	before	15.45	33.75	11.924	0.001
	during	31.87	50.01		

In contrast, analysis of the male group related differences in body variables, and those related to sexual arousal and anxiety, before and during the lockdown, showed no quantitative or qualitative changes to any of the variables considered (See Table 3).

Table 3. Comparison of body variables and sexual arousal and anxiety before and during the lockdown in men.

Men's Scores (n = 140)		Mean	Std. Deviation	F	Sig
Weight Phobia	before	1.2	1.1	0.142	0.707
	during	1.3	1.5		
Body Image Concern	before	1.1	1.1	0.006	0.938
	during	1.1	1.5		
Avoidance	before	0.7	1.1	0.471	0.493
	during	0.8	1.4		
Compulsive self-monitoring	before	1.0	0.9	0.314	0.575
	during	1.1	1.4		
Depersonalization	before	0.7	1.1	1.347	0.247
	during	0.9	1.5		
Global Severity Index	before	1.0	1.0	0.223	0.637
	during	1.1	1.4		
Sexual Arousability	before	125.53	29.82	0.296	0.587
	during	123.16	42.10		
Sexual Anxiety	before	35.86	60.39	1.264	0.262
	during	43.82	58.10		

3.3. Correlations

To further investigate the results that emerged, and (H2) to test the correlations between the different variables before and during lockdown, statistical correlation analyses were used in the female sample for both pre-lockdown and lockdown data.

Table 4 shows the correlations between body experience and sexual experience before lockdown in women. After Bonferroni correction, a p value of 0.006 was considered statistically significant. It should be noted that the subscales of the BUT show a strong internal correlation. Other significant correlations included:

- a negative correlation between weight phobia and age,
- a positive, but weak, correlation between compulsive self-image checks and sexual arousal,
- a positive correlation between depersonalization and sexual anxiety.

Table 4. Correlations between body image dimensions, arousal, and sexual anxiety in women before lockdown.

	Weight Phobia	BIC	AV	CSM	DEP	GSI	Sex Arous.	Sex Anx
BIC-Body Image Concern	0.892 **							
AV-Avoidance	0.718 **	0.812 **						
CSM-Compulsive self-monitoring	0.803 **	0.780 **	0.733 **					
DEP-Depersonalization	0.676 **	0.752 **	0.882 **	0.737 **				
GSI-Global Severity Index	0.928 **	0.955 **	0.892 **	0.883 **	0.861 **			
Sexual Arousability	−0.039	0.033	0.104	0.161 *	0.104	0.061		
Sexual Anxiety	0.021	0.087	0.153	0.131	0.167 *	0.108	0.131	
Age	−0.171 *	−0.151	−0.065	−0.111	−0.081	−0.139	−0.027	0.000

Legend: Correlation is significant at ** 0.01 level (2-tailed) * 0.05 level (2-tailed).

Table 5, on the other hand, shows the correlations between body experience and sexual experience in women during the lockdown. Highly significant correlations emerged between variables relating to body image alteration and sexual arousal and anxiety. The function of sexual arousal showed highly significant negative correlations with all parameters concerning body image alteration. In contrast, anxiety related to arousal factors showed highly significant positive correlations with all parameters concerning body image alteration.

Table 5. Correlations between body image size and sexual arousal and anxiety in women during lockdown.

	Weight Phobia	BIC	AV	CSM	DEP	GSI	Sex Arous.	Sex Anx.
BIC-Body Image Concern	0.937 **							
AV-Avoidance	0.840 **	0.892 **						
CSM-Compulsive self-monitoring	0.880 **	0.885 **	0.845 **					
DEP-Depersonalization	0.825 **	0.895 **	0.946 **	0.866 **				
GSI-Global Severity Index	0.953 **	0.977 **	0.942 **	0.937 **	0.942 **			
Sexual Arousability	−0.259 **	−0.273 **	−0.397 **	−0.280 **	−0.403 **	−0.327 **		
Sexual Anxiety	0.578 **	0.626 **	0.668 **	0.600 **	0.688 **	0.657 **	−0.280 **	
Age	−0.193 **	−0.163 *	−0.120	−0.128	−0.088	−0.153	−0.050	−0.114

Legend: Correlation is significant at ** 0.01 level (2-tailed). * 0.05 level (2-tailed).

4. Discussion

The present study investigated the relationship between body image quality and sexual excitability or anxiety before and during the COVID-19 pandemic. The most recent literature [1,2,4] reviewed, showed important alterations in sexual behavior that were independent from gender, geographical region, race, or sexual orientation. There is clear evidence that the lockdown has had an impact on the sexual behavior of millions of people. The theoretical framework on body image explains very well how sexuality is strongly related to body image: the body is a vehicle for the expression of sexuality, and consequently, alterations in self-image can hinder a healthy expression of excitability. We hypothesized that the two factors were related, although there are few studies linking body image and sexual arousability. This study fills a gap in a field of which we only have partial knowledge.

It is well known that body awareness is fundamental to identity, self-esteem, and self-value constructs. Body mediates identification and self-direction processes. Identity definition allows individuals to determine their priorities, to organize goals, and behaviors in a connected and coherent way, to direct actions and efforts effectively, to act consistently with personal values, to be resilient while maintaining levels of well-being and emotional satisfaction. A negative alteration of body image may be reflected in low quality of life and has often been found to underlie psychiatric disorders [27–29]. To date, the body image literature has focused on the relationship between an ideal of thinness and perfection, finding it linked to high rates of body dissatisfaction, as predictive factors for the development of eating disorders and depressive disorders, especially among women.

The impact of the pandemic on sexuality has recently been the subject of several studies. The decrease in arousal, found in the present study, agrees with alterations found in other general population surveys conducted during the lockdown. However, the relationship between these alterations to sex life had not, thus far, been correlated with body image, taking into account gender differences. This makes the results original, but on the other hand, poorly comparable.

Our study showed that gender significantly affects body image perceptions, sexual arousability, and anxiety. In particular, the female sample showed a significant difference (i.e., a negative modification of the relationship with the body during the lockdown phase) compared with the previous period. This worsening phenomenon was also found in sexual arousal related functions and revealed an increase in sexual anxiety.

Interestingly, that sexual experiences were worsening was not valid for the male sample. This finding may underscore a greater predisposition of the female gender to respond to a peculiar situation, albeit a rare one, such as a pandemic lockdown, with bodily discomfort affecting sexual life.

An interesting hypothesis is that the difference between men and women in the perception of their body image, and consequently in their quality of life, is influenced by both sociocultural and neurobiological factors [30,31]. From a neurobiological perspective, anxiety was found in subjects exposed to body image stimuli, and there was an increase in the activation of the amygdala as well as in the anterior cingulate cortex. Plausibly, this activation is the expression of mixed emotions, such as fear and anxiety, in response to negative body image related perceptions. Interestingly, this activation is not detected among males, and only characterized the women's sample. This finding could lead to the hypothesis that the idea of thinness is rooted in a neurological circuit based on an emotional response among women, and this deep activation could be responsible for some aspects of eating and body image disorders [32].

From a socio-cultural perspective, there is a connection between social success and physical appearance, as well as between mental health and satisfaction with body image, especially for women. It has been found that women, compared to men, make more effort and spend more time to realize their ideal social image. In fact, they are more likely to resort to aesthetic surgery, nutritional and dietary counselling, and use more social comparison mechanisms. The most requested cosmetic surgery procedures by women are increase in breast size, followed by fat liposuction on buttocks, abdomen, and thighs, and this may suggest body image concerns [33].

In addition, gender differences are historically notable in terms of eating disorders such as anorexia nervosa and bulimia nervosa [34]. By adolescence, girls may become part of an all-female subculture in which topics of discussion and behaviors are associated with maintaining appearance, with dangerous psychopathological drifts. Recent studies show that adolescent females, given their vulnerable bodily self-esteem, are more likely to affiliate with blogs and groups that promote the development of eating disorders [35–37].

Increasingly, "sexiness" is also part of the ideal image of women. Women, and even adolescent girls, are encouraged to accept a view of sex that legitimizes their role as a sex object. In a study conducted at a college, the female sample reported a detailed list of characteristics that women consider to be fundamental to appear more sexy to men. Females included a range of activities, including shaving armpits, legs, arms, and genitals; wearing short skirts and bras that enhance the shape of the breast; caring and straightening hair; wearing a good perfume and bikini. In contrast, among the sample of young men belonging to the same college, it was found that the majority of men, to appear sexy to women, listed only two characteristics: wearing perfume and being clean [38,39].

Sexual hyper-investment in body image does not correspond to better bodily self-esteem nor sexual satisfaction, quite the contrary. It is important to emphasize that the data analyzed showed an absence of correlations between body experience and sexual arousal in women in the pre-lockdown phase, as opposed to the correlations that emerged in the lockdown period. This result suggests that the alteration of bodily experience in the lockdown phase has modified the experiences of sexual desire and arousal negative for women.

5. Limitations and Conclusions

Some limitations of the study need to be highlighted. The subjects responded to an online survey. Hence, the lack of control by the experimenter could not limit the effects of errors due to possible confounding factors in the subject's environment. The effects of boredom, distraction, and social desirability were not estimated.

The research design involved the dual administration of the same questionnaire. At first, subjects had to respond by thinking about their sexual experience before the lockdown, and then they had to respond again by thinking about their experience during the lockdown. This can generate several limitations, such as the halo effect. Another possible bias could be caused by responding retrospectively to a condition experienced in the past. The ideal condition would have been to detect the sexual experience at least six months earlier. However, no one could have predicted a worldwide pandemic.

It should be also noted that conducting a techno-mediated survey reduces the target population to individuals who own an internet connection and digital devices such as personal computers, tablets, and smartphones. Moreover, most of the sample have high educational qualifications, which reduces the possibility of generalization to different social contexts or backgrounds. However, data collection, as outlined by the *APA in Opportunities and Challenges on Online Psychological Research* [40], was the only possible mode during a time of great restrictions, even for researchers.

The lockdown had complex anthropological, social, and existential implications that are not yet sufficiently known. The pandemic factor, represented for the first time in history through continuous alarmist information from the mass media, has profoundly changed our perception towards the world and the others. Beyond the hypotheses that can be formulated, it appears evident from our preliminary data that women experience their relationships to their bodies and sexualities with greater discomfort.

Although the understanding of this gender difference deserves in-depth studies that necessitate being targeted and interdisciplinary, a contribution that this work is that it can give greater attention to the level of support and psychological assistance that women need at this time in history, and that is expected to continue for a long time.

Government initiatives related to emergency management have included psychological care planning focused on COVID-19 positive patients, and health care workers undergoing severe stress and traumatic experiences. However, the need for the psychological support of the general population has not been fully realized.

The results of this study highlight that psychological support represents a central, albeit underestimated, health factor. Particular attention should be directed towards the female population, since some aspects of mental suffering seem to be particularly related to gender.

Psychological interventions should be targeted and specific considering that we are facing a completely new phenomenon that could undermine the psychological balance in the general population, laying the groundwork for future psychopathological expressions that are not predictable.

Author Contributions: C.C. and C.M. conceived the research design. M.C.P., A.R. and F.I. were responsible for data collection and interview dissemination. M.C.P. and A.R. reviewed the literature and drafted the first version of the manuscript. C.C. carried out the statistical analysis. M.R.A.M. and G.P. supervised the project. All authors provided critical feedback and helped shape the research, analysis and approved the final manuscript. All authors have read and agreed to the published version of the manuscript.

Funding: This research received no specific grant from any funding agency in the public, commercial, or not-for-profit sectors.

Institutional Review Board Statement: Not available.

Informed Consent Statement: The School of Psychiatry of Messina University (Italy), is investigating sexual excitability and anxiety associated with body image in relation to the lockdown period for COVID-19 Pandemic. We are interested in how body image-related discomfort, avoidant behaviors and compulsive control may affect people's sexual life. You will be asked to answer short questionnaires. The survey will take about 15 min and respect anonymity and personal information, according to the current privacy law. The collected data will be used only for scientific research purposes. If you are under 18 years, you must ask your parents for consent. If you are taking the survey via cell phone, you will need to put your screen horizontally to view all response options. Thanks for your cooperation.

Data Availability Statement: Not available.

Conflicts of Interest: The authors declare that there is no financial, general, and institutional conflict of interest regarding the publication of this article.

References

1. Arafat, S.Y.; Alradie-Mohamed, A.; Kar, S.K.; Sharma, P.; Kabir, R. Does COVID-19 pandemic affect sexual behaviour? A cross-sectional, cross-national online survey. *Psychiatry Res.* **2020**, *289*, 113050. [CrossRef] [PubMed]
2. Lehmiller, J.J.; Garcia, J.R.; Gesselman, A.N.; Mark, K.P. Less sex, but more sexual diversity: Changes in sexual behavior during the COVID-19 coronavirus pandemic. *Leis. Sci.* **2021**, *43*, 295–304. [CrossRef]
3. Coombe, J.; Kong, F.Y.S.; Bittleston, H.; Williams, H.; Tomnay, J.; Vaisey, A.; Hocking, J.S. Love during lockdown: findings from an online survey examining the impact of COVID-19 on the sexual health of people living in Australia. *Sexually Transm. Infect.* **2021**, *97*, 357–362. [CrossRef] [PubMed]
4. Li, G.; Tang, D.; Song, B.; Wang, C.; Qunshan, S.; Xu, C.; Geng, H.; Wu, H.; He, X.; Cao, Y. Impact of the COVID-19 Pandemic on Partner Relationships and Sexual and Reproductive Health: Cross-Sectional, Online Survey Study. *J. Med. Internet Res.* **2020**, *22*, e20961. [CrossRef]
5. Jacob, L.; Smith, L.; Butler, L.; Barnett, Y.; Grabovac, I.; McDermott, D.; Armstrong, N.; Yakkundi, A.; Tully, M.A. Challenges in the Practice of Sexual Medicine in the Time of COVID-19 in the United Kingdom. *J. Sex. Med.* **2020**, *17*, 1229–1236. [CrossRef] [PubMed]
6. Otero, M.C.; Fernández, M.L.; Castro, Y.R. Influencia de la imagen corporal y la autoestima en la experiencia sexual de estudiantes universitarias sin trastornos alimentarios. *Int. J. Clin. Health Psychol.* **2004**, *4*, 357–370.
7. Cash, T.F. *Body Image: A Handbook of Science, Practice, and Prevention*; Smolak, L., Ed.; Guilford Press: New York, NY, USA, 2011.
8. Tiggemann, M. Body image across the adult life span: Stability and change. *Body Image* **2004**, *1*, 29–41. [CrossRef]
9. Tylka, T.L.; Wood-Barcalow, N.L. What is and what is not positive body image? Conceptual foundations and construct definition. *Body Image* **2015**, *14*, 118–129. [CrossRef] [PubMed]
10. Posavac, S.S.; Posavac, H.D. Predictors of women's concern with body weight: The roles of perceived self-media ideal discrepancies and self-esteem. *Eat. Disord.* **2002**, *10*, 153–160. [CrossRef] [PubMed]
11. Dittmar, H. How do "body perfect" ideals in the media have a negative impact on body image and behaviors? Factors and processes related to self and identity. *J. Soc. Clin. Psychol.* **2009**, *28*, 1–8. [CrossRef]
12. Austin, S.B.; Haines, J.; Veugelers, P.J. Body satisfaction and body weight: Gender differences and sociodemographic determinants. *BMC Public Health* **2009**, *9*, 1–7. [CrossRef] [PubMed]
13. Jones, B.A.; Haycraft, E.; Murjan, S.; Arcelus, J. Body dissatisfaction and disordered eating in trans people: A systematic review of the literature. *Int. Rev. Psychiatry* **2016**, *28*, 81–94. [CrossRef] [PubMed]
14. Jackson, K.L.; Janssen, I.; Appelhans, B.M.; Kazlauskaite, R.; Karavolos, K.; Dugan, S.A.; Avery, E.A.; Shipp-Johnson, K.J.; Powell, L.H.; Kravitz, H.M. Body image satisfaction and depression in midlife women: The Study of Women's Health Across the Nation (SWAN). *Arch. Women's Ment. Health* **2014**, *17*, 177–187. [CrossRef] [PubMed]
15. Etu, S.F.; Gray, J.J. A preliminary investigation of the relationship between induced rumination and state body image dissatisfaction and anxiety. *Body Image* **2010**, *7*, 82–85. [CrossRef]
16. Granillo, T.; Jones-Rodriguez, G.; Carvajal, S.C. Prevalence of eating disorders in Latina adolescents: Associations with substance use and other correlates. *J. Adolesc. Health* **2005**, *36*, 214–220. [CrossRef] [PubMed]
17. Furnham, A.; Badmin, N.; Sneade, I. Body image dissatisfaction: Gender differences in eating attitudes, self-esteem, and reasons for exercise. *J. Psychol.* **2002**, *136*, 581–596. [CrossRef] [PubMed]
18. McGuinness, S.; Taylor, J.E. Understanding body image dissatisfaction and disordered eating in midlife adults. *N. Z. J. Psychol.* **2016**, *45*, 4–12.
19. Peplau, L.A.; Frederick, D.A.; Yee, C.; Maisel, N.; Lever, J.; Ghavami, N. Body image satisfaction in heterosexual, gay, and lesbian adults. *Arch. Sex. Behav.* **2009**, *38*, 713–725. [CrossRef]
20. Paredes, J.; Pinto, B. Imagen corporal y satisfacción sexual. *Ajayu Órgano De Difusión Científica Del Dep. De Psicol. UCBSP* **2009**, *7*, 28–47.
21. Fernández-Bustos, J.G.; González-Martí, I.; Contreras, O.; Cuevas, R. Relación entre imagen corporal y autoconcepto físico en mujeres adolescentes. *Rev. Latinoam. De Psicol.* **2015**, *47*, 25–33. [CrossRef]
22. Body Image, Body Dissatisfaction and Disordered Eating in Relation to Gender and Gender Identity. Available online: http://www.doria.fi/handle/10024/745462012 (accessed on 25 November 2021).
23. Brennan, M.A.; Lalonde, C.E.; Bain, J.L. Body image perceptions: Do gender differences exist? *Psi Chi J. Psychol. Res.* **2010**, *15*, 130–138. [CrossRef]
24. Dang, S.S.; Northey, L.; Dunkley, C.R.; Rigby, R.A.; Gorzalka, B.B. Sexual anxiety and sexual beliefs as mediators of the association between attachment orientation with sexual functioning and distress in university men and women. *Can. J. Hum. Sex.* **2018**, *27*, 21–32. [CrossRef]
25. Cuzzolaro, M.; Vetrone, G.; Marano, G.; Battacchi, M.W. BUT, Body Uneasiness Test: A new attitudinal body image scale. *Psichiatr. Dell'infanzia E Dell'adolescenza* **1999**, *66*, 417–428.
26. Hoon, E.F.; Chambles, D.L. *Sexual Arousability Inventory (SAI) and Sexual Aropusability Inventory-Expanded (SAI-E)*; Graphic Publishing Co: Syracuse, NY, USA, 1986.
27. Rizzo, A.; Bruno, A.; Torre, G.; Mento, C.; Pandolfo, G.; Cedro, C.; Laganà, A.S.; Granese, R.; Zoccali, R.A.; Muscatello, M.R.A. Subthreshold psychiatric symptoms as potential predictors of postpartum depression. *Health Care Women Int.* **2021**, *43*, 129–141. [CrossRef]

28. Mento, C.; Le Donne, M.; Crisafulli, S.; Rizzo, A.; Settineri, S. BMI at early puerperium: Body image, eating attitudes and mood states. *J. Obstet. Gynaecol.* **2017**, *37*, 428–434. [CrossRef] [PubMed]
29. Rizzo, A. Temperament and generativity during the life span. *Mediterr. J. Clin. Psychol.* **2013**, *1*. [CrossRef]
30. Micò, U.; Scimeca, G.; Bruno, A.; Pandolfo, G.; Romeo, V.M.; Mallamace, M.; Zoccali, R.; A Muscatello, M.R. The relationship between personality and sexual motivation: an investigation based on Cloninger's model in nonclinical Italian subjects. *Riv. Di Psichiatr.* **2013**, *48*, 307–314.
31. Scimeca, G.; Bruno, A.; Pandolfo, G.; Micò, U.; Romeo, V.M.; Abenavoli, E.; Schimmenti, A.; Zoccali, R.; Muscatello, M.R.A. Alexithymia, negative emotions, and sexual behavior in heterosexual university students from Italy. *Arch. Sex. Behav.* **2012**, *42*, 117–127. [CrossRef]
32. Friederich, H.-C.; Uher, R.; Brooks, S.; Giampietro, V.; Brammer, M.; Williams, S.C.; Herzog, W.; Treasure, J.; Campbell, I.C. I'm not as slim as that girl: Neural bases of body shape self-comparison to media images. *Neuroimage* **2007**, *37*, 674–681. [CrossRef]
33. Dunkley, C.R.; Brotto, L.A. Disordered Eating and Body Dissatisfaction Associated with Sexual Concerns in Undergraduate Women. *J. Sex Marital. Ther.* **2021**, *47*, 460–480. [CrossRef]
34. Striegel-Moore, R.H.; Bulik, C.M. Risk factors for eating disorders. *Am. Psychol.* **2007**, *62*, 181. [CrossRef] [PubMed]
35. Ramos Valverde, P.; Rivera de los Santos, F.; Moreno Rodríguez, M.D.C. Diferencias de sexo en imagen corporal, control de peso e Índice de Masa Corporal de los adolescentes españoles. *Psicothema* **2010**, *22*, 77–83. [PubMed]
36. Mento, C.; Silvestri, M.C.; Muscatello, M.R.A.; Rizzo, A.; Celebre, L.; Cedro, C.; Zoccali, R.A.; Navarra, G.; Bruno, A. The role of body image in obese identity changes post bariatric surgery. *Eat. Weight Disord.-Stud. Anorex. Bulim. Obes.* **2021**, 1–10. [CrossRef]
37. Mento, C.; Silvestri, M.; Muscatello, M.; Rizzo, A.; Celebre, L.; Praticò, M.; Zoccali, R.; Bruno, A. Psychological Impact of Pro-Anorexia and Pro-Eating Disorder Websites on Adolescent Females: A Systematic Review. *Int. J. Environ. Res. Public Health* **2021**, *18*, 2186. [CrossRef] [PubMed]
38. Calogero, R.M.; Thompson, J.K. Potential implications of the objectification of women's bodies for women's sexual satisfaction. *Body Image* **2009**, *6*, 145–148. [CrossRef] [PubMed]
39. Claudat, K.; Warren, C.S.; Durette, R.T. The relationships between body surveillance, body shame, and contextual body concern during sexual activities in ethnically diverse female college students. *Body Image* **2012**, *9*, 448–454. [CrossRef] [PubMed]
40. Psychological Research Online: Opportunities and Challenges. Available online: https://www.apa.org/science/leadership/bsa/internet/internet-report (accessed on 25 November 2021).

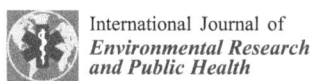

Article

HAPPY MAMA Project (Part 2)—Maternal Distress and Self-Efficacy: A Pilot Randomized Controlled Field Trial

Alice Mannocci [1,*], Sara Ciavardini [2], Federica Mattioli [2], Azzurra Massimi [2], Valeria D'Egidio [2], Lorenza Lia [2], Franca Scaglietta [2], Andrea Giannini [3], Roberta Antico [2,4], Barbara Dorelli [2], Alessandro Svelato [4], Luigi Orfeo [5], Pierluigi Benedetti Panici [3], Antonio Ragusa [4], Giuseppe La Torre [2] and HAPPY MAMA Group [2,†]

1. Faculty of Economics, Mercatorum University, 00186 Rome, Italy
2. Department of Public Health and Infectious Diseases, Sapienza University, 00185 Rome, Italy; saraciavardini@gmail.com (S.C.); mattioli.federica@aslto5.piemonte.it (F.M.); azzurra.massimi@uniroma1.it (A.M.); v.degidio@sanita.it (V.D.); lorenza.lia@uniroma1.it (L.L.); f.scaglietta@gmail.com (F.S.); Robantico76@gmail.com (R.A.); barbara.dorelli@uniroma1.it (B.D.); giuseppe.latorre@uniroma1.it (G.L.T.); alice.mannocci@uniroma1.it (H.M.G.)
3. Department of Maternal and Child Health and Urological Sciences, Umberto I Teaching Hospital, Sapienza University, 00185 Rome, Italy; andrea.giannini@uniroma1.it (A.G.); pierluigi.benedettipanici@uniroma1.it (P.B.P.)
4. Department of Obstetrics and Gynecology, San Giovanni Calibita Fatebenefratelli Hospital, 00186 Rome, Italy; alessandrosvelato@virgilio.it (A.S.); antonio.ragusa@fbf-isola.it (A.R.)
5. Neonatal Intensive Care Unit, "San Giovanni Calibita" Fatebenefratelli, 00186 Rome, Italy; luigi.orfeo@fbf-isola.it
* Correspondence: alice.mannocci@unimercatorum.it
† HAPPY MAMA Group is provided in the Acknowledgments.

Abstract: Introduction: The aim of the pilot randomized controlled field trial is to assess if a midwifery intervention is able to increase the maternal self-efficacy and reduce the stress level during the first six months after birth. Methods: The study was conducted in two different hospitals in Rome, Italy, involving women delivering at or beyond term, aged >18 years old and with normal APGAR scores of the infant. The participants were randomly divided into two groups: "*Individual Intervention Group*" (they received home midwifery assistance for one month after birth, I) and the "*Control Group*" (C). A self-administered questionnaire was administered four times: at the baseline about one week after the hospital delivery (T0), after the intervention about one month after the delivery (T1), and at three months (T2) and at six months after birth (T3). The questionnaire included different validated scales needed to assess maternal perceived self-efficacy (KPCS), parental stress scale stress (PSS) and maternal depressive risk symptoms (EPDS). Results: The study population counted 51 mothers: 28 women in the "C" group and 23 women in the "I" group. The PSS score was statistically higher in the "C" than "I" group at T1 ($p = 0.024$); whereas the KPCS score was statistically higher in the "I" ($p = 0.039$) group; EPDS score did not show significant difference between the two groups in the follow-up period. An inverse significant correlation between KPCS and PSS was found during the study window time ($p < 0.0001$). Conclusions: These results potentially give the opportunity to explore this area of focus further, in order to better address maternal individual needs for the successful transition to motherhood. More research in this area is required.

Keywords: self-efficacy; mindfulness; stress; post-partum; newborn; mother-infant; maternal behavior; mother-infant interaction; maternal parenting stress; maternal support

1. Introduction

In spite of the popular saying that women have a maternal instinct, the postpartum period is a time very commonly accompanied by anxiety, uncertainties, and fear [1]. Women have to quickly adapt to a new routine and face new responsibilities and tasks, such as breastfeeding, which can be challenging for a primiparous mother. The period after birth is often characterized by changes in sleeping habits, family dynamics, but also changes in the woman's body, and as the presence of several physical health conditions, have been found in the two years postpartum [1–3]. These can cause distress and fatigue in a new mother, which can be aggravated in case of lack of social support and a sound financial condition [4].

Until now, research on this topic has focused on postpartum depression [5] while postpartum maternal health was often neglected [6,7]. Considering that the stress and other psychological conditions during this period can have negative consequences for the mother and the baby [8], research in the area of psychological suffering during the period after birth is needed.

But why should a new mother be stressed out? This may occur when a new mother perceives that responsibilities exceed her available coping resources, and thus she will experience stress [9], and chronic stress can result in mental health problems [10].

For this reason, it should be taken into consideration that during the postpartum period, the motherhood can be supported by health interventions that give support and information [8,11].

For assessing the efficacy of the interventions that focused on the increase of wellbeing and reduction of anxiety, stress and depression should be monitored. Mindfulness and self-efficacy [12] are considered key elements in influencing pain intensity, daily functioning, decision-making and the ability to self-regulate and control personal destiny [13].

What are self-efficacy and mindfulness in motherhood?

Self-efficacy refers to an individual's' beliefs in their ability to successfully perform specific behaviors needed to function effectively in a particular domain [14–16]. When contextualizing self-efficacy in the parental domain, it is referred to as maternal parental self-efficacy (MPSE) [17]. The MPSE encompasses both the level of perceived knowledge of appropriate child-rearing behaviors and the degree of confidence in one's ability to perform parenting tasks. For a mother to perceive herself as efficacious in parenting, she must have (a) a repertoire of responses to typical child-rearing situations (e.g., methods of soothing a crying infant, ways to manage a toddler's disruptive behavior), (b) confidence in her ability to carry out these interventions, (c) beliefs that her child will respond to her efforts, and (d) beliefs that significant others will support her efforts [18,19]. It is the cognitive belief mothers hold in their ability to perform newborn-care tasks, and it is one of the most crucial components for the smooth transition to motherhood [20–22].

Mindfulness is the awareness that emerges when we learn to pay deliberate and wholehearted attention to the moment-by-moment unfolding of the external and internal world [23]. Consequently, the mindfulness-based interventions (MBIs) have been identified as stress-reducing and psychological improvement enhancers [24]. In the context of pregnancy and motherhood, a recent systematic review and meta-analysis of mindfulness-based interventions in pregnancy found that mindfulness-based interventions may be beneficial for outcomes such as anxiety, depression, perceived stress and levels of mindfulness [25]. Similarly, a systematic review of the effectiveness of MBIs on maternal perinatal mental health outcomes offered preliminary evidence for the effectiveness of the interventions in reducing anxiety [26].

A pilot study showed that mothers that received a MBIs in the perinatal and postpartum period reported significantly higher maternal self-efficacy, mindfulness components, and self-compassion than those in the control group, and also reported lower anxiety, stress, and psychological distress [27].

Another qualitative study has revealed that women often feel the need for help after delivery [28]. Evidence from Finland has shown that breastfeeding is eased and continued due to the mother's resources and attitude to breastfeeding, support from her social network, and the current promotion of breastfeeding in society [29] which could be increased by interventions that give support and information to women.

The purpose of the present pilot study is to assess if an intervention focused to increase the maternal well-being and self-efficacy of Italian women during the first six months after childbirth prevents or reduces stress levels and the risk of depression. The main hypothesis of the study is that women with higher level of maternal self-efficacy experience lower levels of stress.

This study aims to engage and empower new mothers by strengthening their parenting skills. High parental confidence predicts several parental and child outcomes [30] and act as a protective factor against maternal depression, stress, relationship difficulties and compromised child development [1]. The conceptual framework underlying the intervention is Bandura's self-efficacy theory: self-efficacy is defined as "the belief in one's capabilities to achieve a goal or perform a task and can influence personal motivation and ability to succeed" [15,31]. This approach was widely used for health promotion and to obtain behavioral changes in several contexts and in different kinds of patients. In this specific context, parental self-efficacy is defined as "the beliefs or judgments a parent holds of their capabilities to organize and execute a set of tasks related to parenting a child" [32]. Parental efficacy could also be defined as "the parent's beliefs in his or her ability to influence the child and his or her environment to foster the child's development and success" [14].

Therefore, the HAPPY MAMA intervention is globally focused on the mother-child dyad and aims to teach both the basic elements for effective childcare and behavioral strategies to cope with the difficulties that occur during this period.

2. Methods

2.1. Design of the Study

A randomized controlled field trial was carried out in two Italian hospitals of Rome, Italy. The CONSORT statement was followed to perform the research [33,34].

2.1.1. Ethical Approval and Registration of the Protocol

Ethics approval for the full study was obtained (Protocol number 826/19, RIF.CE: 5559, date 12 September 2019). The protocol of the study was registered on the Clinicaltrials.gov database (accessed on 8 November 2021, ID number: 80209930587).

2.1.2. Eligibility Criteria for Participants

The following eligibility criteria were applied: only women aged 18 years old or older and who were able to communicate in Italian were enrolled.

The following exclusion criteria were applied:

(1) women were excluded from the study if they or their babies had serious health problems;
(2) gestational age ≤37 weeks, weight of the baby <2500 g [35];
(3) APGAR score <7 immediately after birth [36].

Participants with whose criteria did not match those listed above were excluded from the study, as these might influence the outcomes [22,37] and pose a threat to the internal validity of the study.

Participants were recruited from the Obstetrics Units of the hospitals.

For organizational reasons, only mothers who live in the city of Rome were enrolled.

The enrollment of participants was conducted from 0 to three days postpartum by the researchers and research nurses using a brochure explaining the aim of the study.

The recruitment period was three months (October–December 2019). Prior to study participation, all women who agreed to participate were asked to sign a written consent form and to provide a contact phone number and e-mail.

2.1.3. Randomization and Blinding

After obtaining the informed consent, the mothers were divided into two groups: the "individual intervention group", called "IG", and the "control group", called "CG". The CG received routine care only. This care involved postnatal support by nurses and midwives in the hospital and a follow-up (around one to six weeks post-delivery) via an outpatient appointment with the doctor at the hospital.

All women recruited were randomly allocated to the groups. Simple randomization was realized using a random number sequence generated with Epicalc 2000. For equal allocation to the two groups, odd and even numbers were used to indicate treatments I and C, respectively. The groups were matched according to the following variables:

1. age (>34 years, 34 is the mean age of Italian women at childbirth) [38];
2. vaginal delivery (Yes/No).

These variables are considered in the randomization because the literature has highlighted a causal link with stress levels [38,39].

Four groups were created for allocation: age >34 and vaginal delivery; age >34 and no vaginal delivery; age ≤34 and vaginal delivery; age ≤34 and no vaginal delivery. The random number was associated to one group on the basis of the residue class modulo 4: the least residue system modulo 4 is {0, 1, 2, 3}.

2.2. Data Collection

The recruitment lasted two weeks. During the delivery, a researcher requested that each participant sign consent forms and then collected the demographic information for matching and performing the randomization.

During this preliminary phase, a unique code was assigned to each woman.

For organizational reasons, one researcher had a paper sheet that reported the codes associated to the women's names. After the recruitment and the randomization phase a data collection phase was started.

A message that contains the link to the questionnaire and the personal code was sent by phone. The personal code was used to identify the on-line questionnaires and preserve the anonymity of the participants.

The questionnaire was created using Google Forms and administered online four times:

1. At T0: about one week after the hospital delivery;
2. At T1: about one months after the delivery and after the home intervention;
3. At T2: three months after the delivery;
4. At T3: six months after the delivery.

2.3. Questionnaire

An online questionnaire was used to obtain socio-demographic data including age, civil status (single or not), employment (student/worker/no worker), educational level (middle school/high school/university), ethnicity, *the birth date*, primiparous (yes/no), the number of children living at home, and age, vaginal birth (yes/no), and characteristics of breastfeeding practice.

The questionnaire adopted for data collection was composed by three validated scales:

1. The Karitane Parenting Confidence Scale (KPCS) [40] was used. More precisely, the Italian version (KPCS-IT) validated by Mannocci et al. was included [41]. The KPCS scale measures perceived parental self-efficacy (PPSE), which is defined as "beliefs or judgments a parent holds of their capabilities to organize and execute a set of tasks related to parenting a child" [42]. The 15-item scale, based on self-efficacy theory [15], was developed to assess the PPSE of parents with infants aged 0–12 months. The factor analysis has revealed a three-factor structure: efficacy, support, and child development. This 15-item questionnaire was scored on a five-point Likert scale, where 0 = No, hardly ever; 1 = No, not very often; 2 = Yes, some of the time; 3 = Yes, most of the time). The internal consistency of the questionnaires KPCS-IT was estimated as 0.801 [41].
2. The Parental Stress Scale (PSS) [42] was used; more precisely, the Italian version (PSS-IT) validated by Mannocci et al. [41]. The PSS scale consisted of 18 items rated on a 5-point Likert scale (1 = low agree/5 = strong agree) The total score was obtained by summing up the value for each item. A higher score indicates a higher level of parental stress. The internal consistency of the PSS-IT studied by Mannocci et al. reported a Cronbach's alpha = 0.862 [41].

3. The Italian version of the Edinburgh Postnatal Depression Scale (EPDS) [43–45]. The EPDS version published by Benvenuti et al. [43] is used to measure maternal depressive symptoms. The EPDS is a self-report screening measure used to detect symptoms of postpartum depression. Scores >12 on the EPDS are correlated with a diagnosis of major depressive disorder (MDD) [46].

During the administration of the follow-up questionnaires (T1, T2 and T3), the section on socio-demographic variables was removed.

2.4. HAPPY MAMA Intervention

2.4.1. Personnel Involved in the Intervention

The health care workers involved in the administration of the interventions consisted of midwives, nurses, job-infant care workers and students in obstetrics who acted as tutors during the interventions.

2.4.2. Intervention

A training course was carried out by a childcare worker and a midwife with high experience in childcare and home interventions. The participants in the training course were the operators that were involved in the administration of the intervention for the "IG". The HAPPY MAMA intervention includes educational and mindfulness training and simulations of typical events. Given the importance of communication skills training and better outcomes in studies where skills practice has taken place, the interventionists developed their skills through patient simulations and role-play scenarios with one another and with the facilitators before interacting with study participants.

Objectives

The objective of the HAPPY MAMA intervention is to improve the maternal self-efficacy and mood control. In other words, it is to offer supports and techniques to increase confidence and to reduce stress. In particular, the first goal is to make new mothers recognize their abilities and to increase self-awareness: control and self-management are important for the process of learning mindfulness and with regard to the ability to care for the baby; the second one is to put new mothers in a condition to implement strategies and techniques practically in order to pursue goals to restore mental well-being.

Structure

The HAPPY MAMA intervention finds analogies and inspirations in problem-solving training [47]. The problem solving training is a therapeutic intervention, used if the gambler shows poor problem solving skills when coping with excessive gambling activities. A therapist usually introduces a problem solving technique [48] that involves the following five steps: (i) defining the problem, (ii) collecting information about the problem, (iii) generating different solutions, (iv) listing advantages and disadvantages for each solution, and (v) implementing and evaluating the solution. According to this approach, the intervention was thought and planned as follows:

1. Listening and establishing relationship phases

The first step is characterized by listening and understanding the critical points from the new mother. This requires the use of listening skills, empathy, authenticity, and acceptance. The operator maintains a nonjudgmental approach and allows the woman to determine the need for behavioral change, rather than offering unsolicited advice on the need for change.

2. Analysis of the problems

The situation has to be carefully evaluated, considering the discomfort and emotional distress involved. The stress situation is described in a subjective way, from the new mother, and she will assign a grade of discomfort for each problem.

3. Assessment

The operator will carry out a multidimensional evaluation of the mother within the dyad. The operator will evaluate the strategies implemented by the new mother to face problems and difficulties, for example: how she routinely handles organizational problems, how she experiences breastfeeding if there is a lack of sleep, and how she considers her family and support network.

The evaluation will have to consider the environment as a whole, with attention to facilitators and barriers.

4. Definition of the problem and the goal of the intervention

The problems detected by the operator may be explained and summarized to the participants. The operator only explores ways to implement change once the woman expresses the desire and confidence to change.

The shared identification of the mothers' priority will lead to the definition of a tailored plan aimed at achieving specific goals such as the reduction of the stress levels, the reduction in sleep deprivation (hours of sleep per night), optimization of breastfeeding (number, duration and quality), and increased well-being (mental health, physical health).

Strategies of concrete action and planned behavior have to be adapted to the context and to the mother's coping style. The length of the intervention is about three hours in one day.

2.4.3. Sample Size

The method of setting the pilot trial sample size was applied [49,50], and the following parameters were chosen to establish the sample size:

1. average depression score measured with EPDS after childbirth is equal to mean = 5.1 and SD = 2.96 [43];
2. hypothesis: SD is similar in the "IG" and the standardized difference (effect size) of EPDS will be $0.1 \leq d \leq 0.3$ (small effect) [49], namely that the EPDS mean in the IG was lower $4.2 \leq$ mean EPDS ≤ 4.8. The hypothesis of a small effect size was chosen because it is the first time that the HAPPY MAMA intervention was carried out and the effects are unknown. The small effect observed in the literature for other similar interventions was also considered [27,51];
3. the level of significance and power of the study are 95% and 80%, respectively.

On account of these parameters, the pilot sample size is $N = 20$ for each group.

An increment of 20% for possible missing data and lost to the follow-up was considered. A total of 48 women (24 women for each group), were recruited.

2.5. Statistical Methods

Pre-protocol analysis was adopted: the sample included only those patients who completed the treatment originally allocated at different times.

Descriptive statistics was used to show the characteristics of the sample and to analyze the feasibility and acceptability of the study protocol. Measures of central tendency (mean and median) and variability (Standard Deviation, SD, and minimum and maximum) for continuous variables and frequencies with percentages for categorical variables were computed.

The outcomes PSS, KPCS, and EPDS were described, stratifying by demographic characteristics and monitored in time periods (T0, T1, T2 and T3).

A univariate analysis was conducted to compare the different groups (IG and CG) versus primary (PSS and KPCS) and secondary outcomes (EPDS): non-parametric tests were applied to assess the possible differences of the scores between the two groups; a Chi-square test was used to determine possible independence between the groups versus categorical variables.

The tests for paired samples were used to assess the possible changes of the stress score during the follow-up of the control and intervention groups (T0 versus T1, T2 and T3).

Moreover, a bivariate analysis was conducted to assess the possible relationship between the three different outcomes. The correlation coefficient was computed using Spearman's coefficient.

The reliability of the questionnaire was assessment by computing the Cronbach's alpha coefficient.

The significance level was set at $p < 0.05$. Data was analyzed using the IBM SPSS Statistics version 25.0 for Windows (SPSS Inc., Chicago, IL, USA).

3. Results

Ninety-one women were considered to be eligible candidates for the study. Forty women refused to participate (response rate of 56%). The study population counted 51 mothers who answered questionnaires at different follow-up periods.

Concerning the group that refused to enter into the trial, it was possible to collect data on age, type of delivery, and civil status. The mean age was not different to the enrolled sample ($p > 0.05$). Half of these women had a vaginal birth and all of them live with a partner enrolled group ($p > 0.05$). The CONSORT flow diagram of the study enrolment is shown in Figure 1.

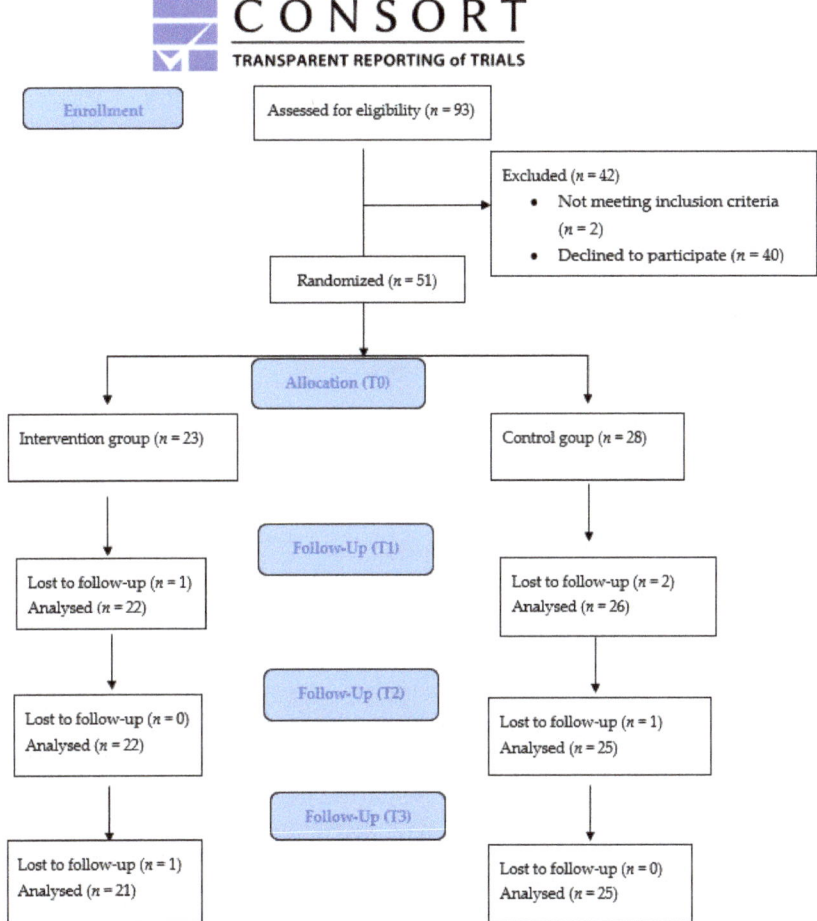

Figure 1. CONSORT flow diagram of the trial.

A total of 28 women were enrolled in the "CG" and 23 women were enrolled in the "IG".

The mothers' characteristics are described in Table 1. The mean age of the sample was 34.3 years old, with a range of 24–44 years old. The majority were graduates, workers, and first-time mothers. All mothers lived with their partners. As for the pregnancy experience, two-thirds of participants had a vaginal birth, according to the national data [52]; women received a different kind of support both during pregnancy and after birth, involving different health care professionals. Mothers adopted various kinds of the newborn feeding, with a high percentage of "Partial breastfeeding" (76.4%), which included both breast milk and formula milk.

Table 1. Characteristics of the sample.

Variables		Total (N = 51)	CG (N = 28)	IG (N = 23)
		N (%)	N (%)	N (%)
Educational level	Middle school	3 (5.9)	1 (3.6)	2 (8.7)
	High school	7 (13.7)	3 (10.7)	4 (17.4)
	University	41 (80.4)	24 (85.7)	17 (73.9)
Employment	Worker	42 (82.3)	26 (92.9)	16 (69.6)
	Housewife	2 (3.9)	0 (0.0)	2 (8.7)
	Student	1 (2.0)	0 (0.0)	1 (4.3)
	No worker	6 (11.8)	2 (7.1)	4 (17.4)
Number of children	1	34 (66.7)	18 (64.3)	16 (69.6)
	2	13 (25.5)	9 (32.1)	4 (17.4)
	>2	4 (7.8)	1 (3.6)	3 (13.0)
Type of birth	Vaginal birth	37 (72.5)	22 (78.6)	15 (65.2)
	Caesarean section	14 (27.5)	6 (21.4)	8 (34.8)
Support received during pregnancy	No	10 (19.6)	6 (21.4)	4 (17.4)
	Yes (Hospital/ASL)	37 (72.6)	19 (67.9)	18 (78.3)
	Yes (Private)	4 (7.8)	3 (10.7)	1 (4.3)
Visits/counselling post-partum	No	33 (64.7)	19 (67.9)	14 (60.9)
	Midwife/childcare	13 (25.5)	7 (25.0)	6 (26.1)
	Clinician	5 (9.8)	2 (7.1)	3 (13.0)
Kind of breastfeeding	Exclusive	11 (21.6)	6 (21.4)	5 (21.7)
	Partial	39 (76.4)	22 (78.6)	17 (74.0)
	No (bottle)	1 (2.0)	0 (0.0)	1 (4.3)
Number of feedings	4–5/day	2 (3.9)	1 (3.6)	1 (4.3)
	6–8/day	31 (60.8)	18 (64.3)	13 (56.6)
	9–10/day	13 (25.5)	6 (21.4)	7 (30.4)
	>10/day	5 (9.8)	3 (10.7)	2 (8.7)

CG: Control Group; IG: Intervention Group; ASL: Azienda Sanitaria Locale (Local Health Unit).

The univariate analysis is described in Table 2. The comparison of the outcomes between the two groups in the different follow-ups was reported.

3.1. KPCS Score

The KPCS score progressively increased in the follow-ups in both groups. A low PPSE (KPCS score < 39) [38] was found at T0 for both groups and at T1 for "CG".

KPCS scores showed a statistically significant difference in the two groups ($p = 0.039$), tat T1 (one month after the individual intervention).

Concerning the reliability of the questionnaire, the Cronbach's alpha at T0 was 0.851.

Table 2. Univariate analysis for the comparison of the KPCS, PSS and EPDS scores between the groups (CG and IG) in the different times of the follow-up.

Variables	(Follow-Up)	CG Mean ± SD Median (Min-Max)	IG Mean ± SD Median (Min-Max)	p *
KPCS	(T0)	35.8 ± 6.0 36.5 (15.0–45.0)	35.0 ± 5.8 35.0 (24.0–44.0)	0.544
	(T1)	37.0 ± 4.9 37.5 (27.0–44.0)	39.7 ± 4.2 41.0 (32.0–45.0)	**0.039**
	(T2)	39.3 ± 3.6 40.0 (32.0–44.0)	39.0 ± 5.6 41.0 (22.0–45.0)	0.614
	(T3)	39.7 ± 4.2 41.0 (28.0–45.0)	40.5 ± 3.8 41.0 (32.0–45.0)	0.458
PSS	(T0)	31.1 ± 6.2 30.0 (21.0–45.0)	34.3 ± 7.5 33.0 (24.0–50.0)	0.105
	(T1)	32.9 ± 9.1 29.5 (22.0–55.0)	27.7 ± 5.6 26.0 (20.0–39.0)	**0.024**
	(T2)	31.1 ± 7.7 30.5 (20.0–51.0)	31.3 ± 9.7 30.0 (18.0–52.0)	0.864
	(T3)	30.1 ± 8.9 28.5 (19.0–54.0)	30.0 ± 8.8 28.0 (18.0–48.0)	0.894
EPDS	(T0)	8.4 ± 4.1 8.0 (0.0–19.0)	8.0 ± 3.2 8.0 (1.0–16.0)	0.924
	(T1)	7.5 ± 4.1 8.0 (0.0–15.0)	6.3 ± 3.5 7.0 (0.0–12.0)	0.246
	(T2)	6.9 ± 3.5 7.0 (1.0–14.0)	6.2 ± 4.2 6.0 (0.0–13.0)	0.575
	(T3)	6.6 ± 5.0 7.0 (0.0–15.0)	6.0 ± 4.8 7.0 (0.0–16.0)	0.575

T0 = one week after delivery; T1 = one month; T2 = three months; T3 = six months. * p-value of Mann-Whitney test. Bold $p < 0.05$. CG: Control Group; IG: Intervention Group; KPCS: Karitane Parenting Confidence Scale; PSS: Parental Stress Scale; EPDS: Edinburgh Postnatal Depression Scale.

3.2. PSS Score

The PSS score has generally been reduced at the end of the follow-ups. The "CG" mean ranged from 30.1(SD = 6.2) at T3 to 32.9 (SD = 9.1) at T1; while the "IG" mean value ranged from 34.3 (SD = 7.5) at T0 to 27.7 (SD = 5.6) at T1. There was not a recommended cut-off (see "Methods" paragraph), but higher scores correlated with higher perceived levels of stress. PSS scores showed a statistically significant difference in the two groups ($p = 0.024$) at two months after birth (T1).

Concerning the reliability of the questionnaire, the Cronbach's alpha at T0 was 0.650.

3.3. EPDS Score

The EPDS score progressively decreased during the follow-ups in both groups, and the recommended cut-off (<12) was reported at all times in both groups.

EPDS scores showed no significant difference ($p > 0.05$) between the two groups in the follow-up.

With regard to the reliability of the questionnaire, the Cronbach's alpha at T0 was 0.754.

The correlation analysis showed an inverse significant correlation between KPCS and PSS over all time: r = −0.464 ($p = 0.001$) at T0, r = −0.621 ($p = 0.000$) at T1, r = −0.598 ($p = 0.000$) at T2 and r = −0.474 ($p = 0.000$) at T3.

4. Discussion

The HAPPY MAMA Project results confirmed the assumption that the postpartum period is one of transition, and new mothers need time to adjust to their new role [53]; PSS, KPCS and EDPS scores improved in the follow-up periods, especially from two to six months postpartum, according to similar evidence [54]. The early postnatal period is characterized by lower maternal confidence (KPCS score < 39), and higher perceived stress (PSS score) and depressive symptoms. It is important to underline that the mentioned scores do not have the purpose of making any particular clinical diagnosis, as the questionnaires were self-administered

Several factors such as changing habits and lack of experience can affect either maternal confidence or mood; these feelings may improve after some weeks, after becoming more skilled and self-confident, as underlined by Kristensen et al. in a similar study [54]. This is also pointed out in the first phase of the HAPPY MAMA Project [41], which shows a strong inverse correlation between KPCS and PSS scores. The review carried out by Alberese et al. also showed a statistically significant inverse correlation between the perceived self-efficacy (PSE) and depression symptoms ($p < 0.05$), therefore at each follow up a better maternal PSE corresponds to lower perceived maternal stress [55]. Concerning the hypothesis of causal connection, that is that the PSE should buffer against stress levels, Albanese et al.'s review confirms that PSE is a key factor affecting both the parent and the child's well-being. On the other hand, reverse causality could be likely too: parents who are more stressed have less resources to cope with their child. Consequently, their parenting is less effective and hence, their parenting self-efficacy is diminished. This alternative interpretation should be in line with several theoretical accounts like the Family Stress Model [56]. In order to understand if there is a causal relationship, it will be important for future longitudinal works to aid in clarifying the directionality of the relationships between PSE and key outcomes, as well as to monitor how these relationships function over time and in varying contexts.

The present study showed a statically significant difference between the PSS and KPCS score of the "IG" and "CG" only at the first follow-up (T1): "I" group showed a higher KPCS score (Median = 41.0) than "C" group (Median = 37.5) two months after birth and one month after individual home intervention; "IG" also showed a lower PSS score (Median = 26.0) than "CG" (Median = 29.5). The HAPPY MAMA intervention is probably "effective" in the short term, although the definition of efficacy is sufficiently restrictive in this study. In fact, it should be possible to investigate other outcomes such as maternal sleep, baby sleep and weight gain. On the other hand, the results can suggest that a more structured or/and longer support (e.i. more than one home visit or telephone call, and/or counselling or educational booklets) in the intervention could be thought too. Since the intervention was proposed for the first time in this research, it is not possible to find very similar studies. Regardless, the results of this study are in line with those obtained in other studies in first-time mothers.

Missler et al. conducted a randomized controlled trial that was to examine the effectiveness of a brief psychoeducational intervention to prevent postpartum parenting stress, to decrease symptoms of depression and anxiety, and to enhance parental well-being and the quality of caregiving behavior [51]. The intervention consisted of a booklet, a video, a home visit, and a telephone call. The primary outcome was parenting stress postpartum measured using a different tool: the Parenting Stress Index [57].

No differences emerged in levels of parenting stress between the intervention and control group over time. Also, there was no effect of the intervention on symptoms of depression and anxiety, nor on the indices of parental wellbeing (satisfaction with the parenting role, self-efficacy, and sleep quality and quantity) [51]. These results are in agreement with the follow-up results of the HAPPY MAMA trial.

Another similar study was published by Shorey et al. [58]. They studied the effectiveness of a postnatal psychoeducation programme in enhancing maternal self-efficacy and social support and reducing postnatal depression among primiparous women. The intervention group received 90-min face-to-face educational sessions during the home visit, an educational booklet and three follow-up telephone calls. The authors used the same tool to measure the depression risk [45], but a different questionnaire for perceived maternal parental self-efficacy [59] was used. The stress level was not considered. Outcomes were measured at three time points: baseline (on the day of discharge between one to three days postpartum), at six weeks postpartum, and at 12 weeks postpartum. Their findings were shown to be effective in enhancing maternal parental self-efficacy and in reducing postnatal depression at six and 12 weeks postpartum.

In another Iranian clinical trial, the effect of pregnancy training classes based on Bandura's self-efficacy theory on postpartum depression and anxiety was studied. In this case the findings showed that pregnancy training classes based on Bandura self-efficacy theory decreased depression and anxiety during the pregnancy and one month after the delivery [14,60]. The results at one month after the delivery showed a similar effect with the HAPPY MAMA intervention, though different outcomes and tools were applied and the training stared before the delivery.

In agreement with some reflections of Missler et al., several factors could have played a role here. First, it is possible that the intervention is effective on other measures that we did not take into account in this study (e.g., observed sensitive responsiveness, infant well-being). Second, the intervention might be more effective for specific groups of parents (i.e., the sample was relatively well-educated, reporting a high educational level). Also, we lack information on the participants' psychosocial history. Finally, it is possible that the intervention has no added value [51].

The study presents several limitations. The first limitation was the different distribution of the educational level in the sample in comparison with the female adult Italian population: 80.4% of the sample were graduates, even if the percentage of Italian graduated women was 22.4% in 2019 [61]. Secondly, in this project the HAPPY MAMA intervention was applied in "healthy" babies and mothers and with a "normal" gestational age; the effect for other criteria of new-mothers could lead to different results.

With regard to the sample size, the results in this small sample must be considered carefully, since the study population cannot be considered representative of the Italian new mother population. This study, however, lays the foundation for a main trial and overall trial. Additionally, the pilot design of the study did not allow one to have a robust conclusion on the effect of the HAPPY MAMA intervention on the maternal self-efficacy at T1, because they might just result from luck due to the alpha error inflation. Regarding the definition and measurement of PSE, the literature identified a need for extensive psychometric evaluation in future work [62].

With regard to pregnancy, the mothers recruited received different supports during the pregnancy and postpartum period (public or private health care, clinicians involved), and this could have indirectly influenced primary outcomes. Although it was not possible from an ethical point of view to prohibit any other support required by women (especially in the "CG"), if needed.

Moreover, from a statistics point of view, the small sample size did not allow for the performing of a multivariate regression model. Consequently, it was not possible to evaluate the simultaneous effect of different independent variables.

Concerning the EPDS measurement, this study considered the international clinical EPDS cut-off >12 [46], while other studies used a clinical EPDS cut-off >8 [54] or >10 [63]. This choice could have underestimated the risk.

In addition, HAPPY MAMA was a one-time home intervention. It was carried out about one month after birth by self-employed health care providers unknown to mothers. Scientific evidence shows that new-mothers need a holistic support earlier than six-weeks postpartum, and one in the first 10 days would have been better [64]. Similarly, more than one visit would have been better, underlying the importance of the continuity of care to build trusting relationships [65–67]: better to talk about "trusted midwife" or "caseload midwifery" [68]. While previously a mother and her child spent five to six days in the maternity ward, now they generally go home after one or two days; the health care system is not organised to keep pace with these changes [69]. Postnatal continuity care and postpartum home visits are important services that can improve maternal coping and confidence, empowering mothers to take care of their children's health and theirs as well, thus preventing any psychological consequences [63]; that is why the World Health Organization (WHO) recommends "Midwife-led continuity-of-care models, in which a known midwife or small group of known midwives supports a woman throughout the antenatal, intrapartum and postnatal continuum" [68]. Finally, while absence of evidence is not evidence of absence, it should also acknowledge the possibility that one session of intervention aimed at providing information is not sufficient to influence parents' levels of distress, wellbeing and their caregiving quality.

On this field a jeopardized situation of activities is present in Italy: in some Italian regions started to adapt health care services to ensure continuity of care through hospitals and territorial (counselling centers) protocols. In 2010, an institutional "state regions agreement" was created in order to support the services and activities for well-functioning midwifery programs [69,70].

Regarding the strengths of the study, the choice of the home visit has been received favorably by the new-mothers. The support offered to the IG group was never refused (no drop-outs) and was appreciated. In addition, the participation rate in the study (at T3) is acceptable in both groups (8% drop-out in IG and 10% in the CG). The pilot fixed sample size was respected.

The missing values in the questionnaire are absent.

5. Conclusions

This pilot experimental trial was inspired by the willingness to investigate the psychological wellness of new-mothers and to analyse the effect of a single midwifery intervention on mothers' health. It showed that maternal confidence, reduction of stress and mood improve in the months ahead of the intervention. The maternal self-efficacy and perceived stress can be positively influenced by health care support, although this study shows mild effects of one-time intervention. There is therefore the need to analyse the topic in order to better highlight maternal needs and to identify which supports, combinations and how many sessions in an intervention ensure successful transition to motherhood. Large overall randomized trials are required to understand which are the most effective interventions in the postpartum period to sustain and increase women's health and the mother-newborn dyad. It is recommended that further research show the effect of blending mindfulness and skills-based prenatal education program on self-efficacy. In fact, the ultimate goal is institute a system to support women after their delivery that is currently missing in Italy.

Author Contributions: Conceptualization, A.M. (Alice Mannocci), F.S., G.L.T.; methodology and randomization A.M. (Alice Mannocci); enrollment A.M. (Alice Mannocci), S.C., F.M, A.M. (Azzurra Massimi), L.L., V.D., R.A., B.D., A.G.; intervention F.S., H.M.G.; data collection and analysis A.M. (Alice Mannocci), S.C., F.M.; supervision: A.M. (Alice Mannocci), G.L.T., P.B.P., A.R., L.O., A.S.; writing—original draft: A.M. (Alice Mannocci), S.C., F.M., A.M. (Azzurra Massimi); Writing—review & editing: A.M. (Alice Mannocci), A.M. (Azzurra Massimi), V.D., G.L.T. All authors have read and agreed to the published version of the manuscript.

Funding: No financial support was received for the present study.

Institutional Review Board Statement: The study was conducted according to the guidelines of the Declaration of Helsinki, and approved by the Ethics Committee of Umberto I Teaching Hospital (Protocol number 826/19, RIF.CE: 5559, date 12 September 2019). The protocol of the study was registered on the Clinicaltrials.gov database (accessed on 8 November 2021, ID number: 80209930587).

Informed Consent Statement: Written informed consent has been obtained from the patient(s) to publish this paper. The informed consent used in the current study are available from the corresponding author on reasonable request.

Data Availability Statement: The datasets used and/or analysed in the current study are available from the corresponding author on reasonable request.

Acknowledgments: We are extremely grateful to all women who took part in the study. The HAPPY MAMA Group is also composed by: Cristina Alibrandi, Daniela Angelo, Ilaria Gallon, Federica Orlando, Verdiana Pontuale, Flavia Ribelli, Francesca Rotelli, Claudia Scaglione, Michela Scollo and Celeste Taucci.

Conflicts of Interest: The authors declare that they have no conflicts of interests.

References

1. Anderson, C.A. The trauma of birth. *Health Care Women Int.* **2017**, *38*, 999–1010. [CrossRef]
2. Hsu, H.-C.; Wickrama, K.A.S. Maternal life stress and health during the first 3 years postpartum. *Women Health* **2017**, *58*, 565–582. [CrossRef]
3. Cheng, C.-Y.; Li, Q. Integrative Review of Research on General Health Status and Prevalence of Common Physical Health Conditions of Women After Childbirth. *Women's Health Issues* **2008**, *18*, 267–280. [CrossRef] [PubMed]
4. Gallagher, L.; Begley, C.; Clarke, M. Determinants of breastfeeding initiation in Ireland. *Ir. J. Med. Sci.* **2015**, *185*, 663–668. [CrossRef]
5. O'Hara, M.W.; McCabe, J.E. Postpartum Depression: Current Status and Future Directions. *Annu. Rev. Clin. Psychol.* **2013**, *9*, 379–407. [CrossRef] [PubMed]
6. Cheng, C.-Y.; Fowles, E.R.; Walker, L.O. Continuing education module: Postpartum maternal health care in the United States: A critical review. *J. Périnat. Educ.* **2006**, *15*, 34–42. [CrossRef] [PubMed]
7. Coates, R.; de Visser, R.; Ayers, S. Not identifying with postnatal depression: A qualitative study of women's postnatal symptoms of distress and need for support. *J. Psychosom. Obstet. Gynecol.* **2015**, *36*, 114–121. [CrossRef] [PubMed]
8. Potharst, E.S.; Aktar, E.; Rexwinkel, M.; Rigterink, M.; Bögels, S.M. Mindful with Your Baby: Feasibility, Acceptability, and Effects of a Mindful Parenting Group Training for Mothers and Their Babies in a Mental Health Context. *Mindfulness* **2017**, *8*, 1236–1250. [CrossRef]
9. Lazarus, R.S.; Folkman, S. Cognitive Theories of Stress and the Issue of Circularity. In *Dynamics of Stress: Physiological, Psychological and Social Perspectives*; Appley, M.H., Trumbull, R., Eds.; Springer: Berlin, Germany, 1986; pp. 63–80. [CrossRef]
10. Lupien, S.J.; McEwen, B.S.; Gunnar, M.R.; Heim, C. Effects of stress throughout the lifespan on the brain, behaviour and cognition. *Nat. Rev. Neurosci.* **2009**, *10*, 434–445. [CrossRef]
11. Bennett, A.E.; Kearney, J.M. Factors Associated with Maternal Wellbeing at Four Months Post-Partum in Ireland. *Nutrients* **2018**, *10*, 609. [CrossRef]
12. Soysa, C.K.; Wilcomb, C.J. Mindfulness, Self-compassion, Self-efficacy, and Gender as Predictors of Depression, Anxiety, Stress, and Well-being. *Mindfulness* **2015**, *6*, 217–226. [CrossRef]
13. Firth, A.M.; Cavallini, I.; Sütterlin, S.; Lugo, R.G. Mindfulness and self-efficacy in pain perception, stress and academic performance. The influence of mindfulness on cognitive processes. *Psychol. Res. Behav. Manag.* **2019**, *12*, 565–574. [CrossRef] [PubMed]
14. Bandura, A. Self-efficacy: Toward a unifying theory of behavioral change. *Adv. Behav. Res. Ther.* **1978**, *1*, 139–161. [CrossRef]
15. Bandura, A. Regulation of cognitive processes through perceived self-efficacy. *Dev. Psychol.* **1989**, *25*, 729–735. [CrossRef]
16. Bandura, A.; Freeman, W.H.; Lightsey, R. Self-Efficacy: The Exercise of Control. *J. Cogn. Psychother.* **1999**, *13*, 158–166. [CrossRef]
17. Leahy-Warren, P.; McCarthy, G. Maternal parental self-efficacy in the postpartum period. *Midwifery* **2011**, *27*, 802–810. [CrossRef]
18. Coleman, P.K.; Karraker, K.H. Maternal self-efficacy beliefs, competence in parenting, and toddlers' behavior and developmental status. *Infant Ment. Health J.* **2003**, *24*, 126–148. [CrossRef]
19. Troutman, B.; Moran, T.E.; Arndt, S.; Johnson, R.F.; Chmielewski, M. Development of parenting self-efficacy in mothers of infants with high negative emotionality. *Infant Ment. Health J.* **2012**, *33*, 45–54. [CrossRef]
20. Leahy-Warren, P. First-time mothers: Social support and confidence in infant care. *J. Adv. Nurs.* **2005**, *50*, 479–488. [CrossRef]
21. Sanders, M.R.; Wooley, M.L. The relationship between maternal self-efficacy and parenting practices: Implications for parent training. *Child Care Health Dev.* **2005**, *31*, 65–73. [CrossRef]
22. Ngai, F.-W.; Chan, S.W.-C.; Ip, W.-Y. Predictors and Correlates of Maternal Role Competence and Satisfaction. *Nurs. Res.* **2010**, *59*, 185–193. [CrossRef] [PubMed]
23. Williams, J.M.G.; Teasdale, J.D.; Segal, Z.V.; Kabat-Zinn, J. *The Mindful way Through Depression: Freeing Yourself from Chronic Unhappiness*; Guilford Press: New York, NY, USA, 2007.
24. Hughes, A.; Williams, M.; Bardacke, N.; Duncan, L.G.; Dimidjian, S.; Goodman, S.H. Mindfulness approaches to childbirth and parenting. *Br. J. Midwifery* **2009**, *17*, 630–635. [CrossRef]
25. Dhillon, A.; Sparkes, E.; Duarte, R.V. Mindfulness-Based Interventions During Pregnancy: A Systematic Review and Meta-analysis. *Mindfulness* **2017**, *8*, 1421–1437. [CrossRef]
26. Shi, Z.; Macbeth, A. The Effectiveness of Mindfulness-Based Interventions on Maternal Perinatal Mental Health Outcomes: A Systematic Review. *Mindfulness* **2017**, *8*, 823–847. [CrossRef] [PubMed]
27. Perez-Blasco, J.; Viguer, P.; Rodrigo, M.F. Effects of a mindfulness-based intervention on psychological distress, well-being, and maternal self-efficacy in breast-feeding mothers: Results of a pilot study. *Arch. Women's Ment. Health* **2013**, *16*, 227–236. [CrossRef] [PubMed]

28. Coates, R.; Ayers, S.; De Visser, R. Women's experiences of postnatal distress: A qualitative study. *BMC Pregnancy Childbirth* **2014**, *14*, 359. [CrossRef]
29. Tarkka, M.; Paunonen, M.; Laippala, P. Factors related to successful breast feeding by first-time mothers when the child is 3 months old. *J. Adv. Nurs.* **1999**, *29*, 113–118. [CrossRef]
30. Jones, T.L.; Prinz, R.J. Potential roles of parental self-efficacy in parent and child adjustment: A review. *Clin. Psychol. Rev.* **2005**, *25*, 341–363. [CrossRef]
31. Coleman, P.K.; Karraker, K.H. Self-Efficacy and Parenting Quality: Findings and Future Applications. *Dev. Rev.* **1998**, *18*, 47–85. [CrossRef]
32. Montigny, F.; Lacharité, C. Perceived parental efficacy: Concept analysis. *J. Adv. Nurs.* **2005**, *49*, 387–396. [CrossRef]
33. Moher, D.; Hopewell, S.; Schulz, K.F.; Montori, V.; Gøtzsche, P.C.; Devereaux, P.J.; Elbourne, D.; Egger, M.; Altman, D.G. CONSORT 2010 Explanation and Elaboration: Updated guidelines for reporting parallel group randomised trials. *BMJ* **2010**, *340*, c869. [CrossRef] [PubMed]
34. Schulz, K.F.; Altman, D.G.; Moher, D. CONSORT 2010 Statement: Updated Guidelines for Reporting Parallel Group Randomized Trials. *Ann. Intern. Med.* **2010**, *152*, 726–732. [CrossRef]
35. Battaglia, F.C.; Lubchenco, L.O. A practical classification of newborn infants by weight and gestational age. *J Pediatr.* **1967**, *71*, 159–163. [CrossRef]
36. Apgar, V. A proposal for a new method of evaluation of the newborn infant. *Curr. Res. Anesth. Analg.* **1953**, *32*, 260–267. [CrossRef]
37. Brown, S.; Lumley, J. Physical health problems after childbirth and maternal depression at six to seven months postpartum. *BJOG: Int. J. Obstet. Gynaecol.* **2000**, *107*, 1194–1201. [CrossRef] [PubMed]
38. Lean, S.C.; Derricott, H.; Jones, R.L.; Heazell, A.E.P. Advanced maternal age and adverse pregnancy outcomes: A systematic review and meta-analysis. *PLoS ONE* **2017**, *12*, e0186287. [CrossRef]
39. Chen, H.-H.; Lai, J.C.-Y.; Hwang, S.-J.; Huang, N.; Chou, Y.-J.; Chien, L.-Y. Understanding the relationship between cesarean birth and stress, anxiety, and depression after childbirth: A nationwide cohort study. *Birth* **2017**, *44*, 369–376. [CrossRef]
40. Crncec, R.; Barnett, B.; Matthey, S. Development of an instrument to assess perceived self-efficacy in the parents of infants. *Res. Nurs. Health* **2008**, *31*, 442–453. [CrossRef]
41. Mannocci, A.; Massimi, A.; Scaglietta, F.; Ciavardini, S.; Scollo, M.; Scaglione, C.; La Torre, G. HAPPY MAMA Project (PART 1). Assessing the Reliability of the Italian Karitane Parenting Confidence Scale (KPCS-IT) and Parental Stress Scale (PSS-IT): A Cross-Sectional Study among Mothers Who Gave Birth in the Last 12 Months. *Int. J. Environ. Res. Public Health* **2021**, *18*, 4066. [CrossRef]
42. Berry, J.O.; Jones, W.H. The Parental Stress Scale: Initial Psychometric Evidence. *J. Soc. Pers. Relatsh.* **1995**, *12*, 463–472. [CrossRef]
43. Benvenuti, P.; Ferrara, M.; Niccolai, C.; Valoriani, V.; Cox, J.L. The Edinburgh Postnatal Depression Scale: Validation for an Italian sample. *J. Affect. Disord.* **1999**, *53*, 137–141. [CrossRef]
44. Carpiniello, B.; Pariante, C.M.; Serri, F.; Costa, G.; Carta, M.G. Validation of the Edinburgh Postnatal Depression Scale in Italy. *J. Psychosom. Obstet. Gynecol.* **1997**, *18*, 280–285. [CrossRef] [PubMed]
45. Cox, J.L.; Holden, J.M.; Sagovsky, R. Detection of postnatal depression. Development of the 10-item Edinburgh Postnatal Depression Scale. *Br. J. Psychiatry J. Ment. Sci.* **1987**, *150*, 782–786. [CrossRef]
46. Jardri, R.; Pelta, J.; Maron, M.; Thomas, P.; Delion, P.; Codaccioni, X.; Goudemand, M. Predictive validation study of the Edinburgh Postnatal Depression Scale in the first week after delivery and risk analysis for postnatal depression. *J. Affect. Disord.* **2006**, *93*, 169–176. [CrossRef] [PubMed]
47. Nezu, A.M.; Nezu, C.M.; D'Zurilla, T.J. *Problem-Solving Therapy: A Treatment Manual*; Springer Publishing Company: New York, NY, USA, 2013.
48. Goldfried, M.R.; Davison, G.C. *Clinical Behavior Therapy*; Holt, Rinehart & Winston: New York, NY, USA, 1976.
49. Bell, M.L.; Whitehead, A.L.; A Julious, S. Guidance for using pilot studies to inform the design of intervention trials with continuous outcomes. *Clin. Epidemiol.* **2018**, *10*, 153–157. [CrossRef] [PubMed]
50. Whitehead, A.L.; Julious, S.A.; Cooper, C.L.; Campbell, M.J. Estimating the sample size for a pilot randomised trial to minimise the overall trial sample size for the external pilot and main trial for a continuous outcome variable. *Stat. Methods Med Res.* **2016**, *25*, 1057–1073. [CrossRef] [PubMed]
51. Missler, M.; Van Straten, A.; Denissen, J.; Donker, T.; Beijers, R. Effectiveness of a psycho-educational intervention for expecting parents to prevent postpartum parenting stress, depression and anxiety: A randomized controlled trial. *BMC Pregnancy Childbirth* **2020**, *20*, 658. [CrossRef] [PubMed]
52. Italian Ministry of Health, Evento nascita, Il Rapporto Con l'analisi Dei Dati CeDAP. 2016. Available online: http://www.salute.gov.it/portale/news/p3_2_1_1_1.jsp?lingua=italiano&menu=notizie&p=dalministero&id=3882 (accessed on 13 March 2021).
53. Italian Ministry of Health. Puerperio. Retrieved. Available online: http://www.salute.gov.it/portale/donna/dettaglioContenutiDonna.jsp?lingua=italiano&id=4481&area=Salute%20donna&menu=nascita (accessed on 13 March 2021).
54. Kristensen, I.H.; Simonsen, M.; Trillingsgaard, T.; Pontoppidan, M.; Kronborg, H. First-time mothers' confidence mood and stress in the first months postpartum. A cohort study. *Sex. Reprod. Health* **2018**, *17*, 43–49. [CrossRef]
55. Albanese, A.M.; Russo, G.R.; Geller, P.A. The role of parental self-efficacy in parent and child well-being: A systematic review of associated outcomes. *Child Care Health Dev.* **2019**, *45*, 333–363. [CrossRef]

56. Masarik, A.S.; Conger, R.D. Stress and child development: A review of the Family Stress Model. *Curr. Opin. Psychol.* **2017**, *13*, 85–90. [CrossRef]
57. Abidin, R. *Parenting Stress Index: Manual*; Pediatric Psychology Press: Charlottesville, VA, USA, 1983.
58. Shorey, S.; Chan, S.W.C.; Chong, Y.S.; He, H.-G. A randomized controlled trial of the effectiveness of a postnatal psychoeducation programme on self-efficacy, social support and postnatal depression among primiparas. *J. Adv. Nurs.* **2015**, *71*, 1260–1273. [CrossRef]
59. Barnes, C.R.; Adamson-Macedo, E. Perceived Maternal Parenting Self Efficacy (PMP S-E) tool: Development and validation with mothers of hospitalized preterm neonates. *J. Adv. Nurs.* **2007**, *60*, 550–560. [CrossRef]
60. Mohammadi, F.; Kohan, S.; Farzi, S.; Khosravi1, M.; Heidari, Z. The effect of pregnancy training classes based on bandura self-efficacy theory on postpartum depression and anxiety and type of delivery. *J. Educ. Health Promot.* **2021**, *10*, 273. [CrossRef]
61. ISTAT. Livelli Di Istruzione E Ritorni Occupazionali. Anno 21019. 2020. Available online: https://www.istat.it/it/files//2020/07/Livelli-di-istruzione-e-ritorni-occupazionali.pdf (accessed on 8 November 2021).
62. Wittkowski, A.; Garrett, C.; Calam, R.; Weisberg, D. Self-Report Measures of Parental Self-Efficacy: A Systematic Review of the Current Literature. *J. Child Fam. Stud.* **2017**, *26*, 2960–2978. [CrossRef]
63. Milani, H.S.; Amiri, P.; Mohseny, M.; Abadi, A.; Vaziri, S.M.; Vejdani, M. Postpartum home care and its effects on mothers' health: A clinical trial. *J. Res. Med. Sci.* **2017**, *22*, 96. [CrossRef] [PubMed]
64. Walker, S.B.; Rossi, D.M.; Sander, T.M. Women's successful transition to motherhood during the early postnatal period: A qualitative systematic review of postnatal and midwifery home care literature. *Midwifery* **2019**, *79*, 102552. [CrossRef] [PubMed]
65. Lambermon, F.; Vandenbussche, F.; Dedding, C.; van Duijnhoven, N. Maternal self-care in the early postpartum period: An integrative review. *Midwifery* **2020**, *90*, 102799. [CrossRef] [PubMed]
66. Spelke, B.; Werner, E. The Fourth Trimester of Pregnancy: Committing to Maternal Health and Well-Being Postpartum. *Rhode Isl. Med. J.* **2018**, *101*, 30–33.
67. Tully, K.P.; Stuebe, A.M.; Verbiest, S.B. The fourth trimester: A critical transition period with unmet maternal health needs. *Am. J. Obstet. Gynecol.* **2017**, *217*, 37–41. [CrossRef]
68. World Health Organization. *WHO Recommendations on Antenatal Care for a Positive Pregnancy Experience*; World Health Organization: Geneva, Switzerland, 2016.
69. Aune, I.; Dahlberg, U.; Haugan, G. Health-promoting influences among Norwegian women following early postnatal home visit by a midwife. *Nord. J. Nurs. Res.* **2018**, *38*, 177–186. [CrossRef]
70. Ministry of Health. Azioni Regionali Su Accordo Percorso Nascita. Available online: http://www.salute.gov.it/portale/donna/dettaglioContenutiDonna.jsp?lingua=italiano&id=4483&area=Salute%20donna&menu=nascita (accessed on 18 April 2018).

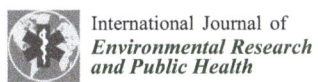

Article

Italian Validation of the Scale of Psychological Abuse in Intimate Partner Violence (EAPA-P)

Giulia Lausi [1,*], Benedetta Barchielli [2], Jessica Burrai [1], Anna Maria Giannini [1] and Clarissa Cricenti [1]

[1] Department of Psychology, Sapienza University of Rome, Via dei Marsi, 00185 Rome, Italy; jessica.burrai@uniroma1.it (J.B.); annamaria.giannini@uniroma1.it (A.M.G.); clarissa.cricenti@uniroma1.it (C.C.)

[2] Department of Dynamic, Clinical Psychology and Health, Sapienza University of Rome, Via degli Apuli, 00185 Rome, Italy; benedetta.barchielli@uniroma1.it

* Correspondence: giulia.lausi@uniroma1.it; Tel.: +39-06-49917534

Abstract: Psychological and emotional forms of violence often represent a danger alarm and an important risk factor for other forms of intimate partner violence (IPV). Measuring psychological violence raises several issues of conceptualization and definition, which lead to the development of several assessment instruments; among them, the Scale of Psychological Abuse in Intimate Partner Violence (EAPA-P) showed good psychometric proprieties in a Spanish population and is used to identify which strategies are acted out to engage in psychological violence. The aim of the present study was to investigate the psychometric properties of the Italian version of EAPA-P among a group of Italian-speaking women (N = 343), thus evaluating its psychometric characteristics. Based on the English translation of the original Spanish version, an 11-item form of the EAPA-P was obtained, validity has been assessed through measures of emotion dysregulation, interpersonal guilt, conflict among partners and depression, anxiety, and stress symptomatology. Moreover, differences among groups were conducted to identify the capacity of the Italian version of EAPA-P to discriminate among women reporting experiencing psychological violence (N = 179), and who don't (N = 150). Results showed an excellent internal validity, good correlations, and a good discriminatory ability of the scale. Strengths, limitations, and practical implications of the study have been discussed according to recent literature.

Keywords: Italian population; psychological violence; self-report; violence against women; gender-based violence; domestic violence; assessment

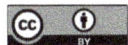

1. Introduction

Intimate partner violence (IPV) is a heterogeneous construct that includes several forms of violence—physical, sexual, economic, psychological/emotional, stalking—perpetrated by an intimate partner [1–3]. Although the reported prevalence of IPV varies considerably across studies [4–9], the findings are in agreement that the prevalence of the emotional/psychological form of violence is higher (5–91%) [5–7,10] than the physical/sexual form (3–59%) [5–7,11,12]. Psychological violence in IPV is frequently experienced in conjunction with other forms of violence, but can also occur alone and precede, or represent an important risk factor for physical/sexual violence [2,13–16].

Given the heterogeneity of IPV, it has been suggested to assess the occurrence of all forms of violence to detect the presence of emotional abuse or coercive control that may represent the first expression of maltreatment in intimate relationships and/or be indicative of a more severe form of IPV [3,17,18]. These considerations underlie the effort made in recent years in studying the consequences of different forms of IPV on women's health. Particularly, several studies [17,19,20] highlighted experiencing psychological violence alone or in conjunction with other forms of violence leads to similar, if not more severe, mental health effects [3,13,21], even after exiting the abusive relationship [22,23].

Psychological violence, either alone or together with other forms of violence, would appear to be closely linked to emotional distress, presence of emotions such as shame and guilt [24–26] and difficulties in emotion regulation [27,28] or symptoms of stress, depression, and anxiety [3,19,22,29–33], suicidal ideation [19,34,35], and lower quality of life [36]. It is worth noting that while mental health effects in terms of psychopathology would seem to be common to all forms of violence, several studies [25,37], although not all of them [38], have found that other effects, such as guilt, would seem to be closely related to psychological abuse and would interact with it by amplifying the possibility of developing psychopathological symptoms such as post-traumatic ones.

1.1. Issues in Defining and Assessing Psychological Violence

Although in recent years there has been a "radical re-evaluation of the importance of emotional abuse in women's mental health" [35,39], one of the reasons underlying the difficulty in comparing studies regarding the prevalence and the effects of psychological violence is based on issues of conceptualization, definition, and measurement of this form of violence [5,17,35,40]. This becomes evident from the use in the literature of broad terminology to refer to psychological violence, often also referred to as emotional abuse, coercion, psychological aggression [2,33,35].

A broad definition of psychological violence has been given by the European Institute for Gender Equality: *"Any act or behavior which causes psychological harm to the partner or former partner. Psychological violence can take the form of, among others, coercion, defamation, a verbal insult or harassment"* ([41], p. 45). Psychological violence is not considered as a unitary construct, but as a form of violence that contains within it several dimensions, such as dominance/isolation and verbal abuse [3,13,17,20,42,43], while other researchers proposed considering psychological violence on a continuum from forms of psychological aggression (e.g., insults) to more intense forms of coercive control [33,44,45]. On the other hand, Marshall [46,47] argued that psychological violence is more than just the dimensions that are identified from time to time, while the most important aspect is the use of the vulnerabilities or strengths of the victim as a weapon in the relationship. In general, the various definitions of psychological abuse include acts such as: yelling or screaming at a partner, insulting, humiliating even in front of other people, harassing, verbally threatening the victim, or loved ones with weapons or without, restricting the victim's access to their social environment, financial resources, vehicle, or telephone, exploiting the victim's vulnerability (e.g., undisclosed sexual orientation) [1,2,5,13,17,32,48,49]. Variations in the terminology and definitions of psychological violence have inevitably been reflected in the psychometric instruments developed to assess this form of violence [3,13,31,33]. Two main limitations of measurement tools in this field are the consideration of psychological violence as a discrete unit [13,17] and the stand-alone assessment of dimensions that fall under psychological violence [33,50,51]. Among the latter instruments are the Dominance Scale-DS [52], which provides a measure of dominance dimensions only. In contrast, most scales in this area are developed for the general measure of IPV or violence against women with a unique measure of the psychological form of violence, such as the Abusive Behavior Inventory [53], the Composite Abuse Scale [54,55], the Index of Psychological Abuse [43,56], the Partner Abuse Scale—Non-Physical [57], the Revised Conflict Tactics Scales (CTS-2) [51,58], the Safe Dates—Psychological Abuse Victimization [59,60], the Women's Experiences with Battering [61–63]. For instance, a major limitation of CTS-2 [51,58], frequently used in studies of psychological violence, is the lack of adequacy and specificity in measuring the construct, not considering psychological violence as a multidimensional construct [31,64,65]. A minority of instruments, on the contrary, have also considered the different dimensions of the construct, such as: the Measure of Wife Abuse [50], which distinguishes between verbal and emotional violence; the Multidimensional Measure of Emotional Abuse [66,67] for measuring restrictive engulfment, hostile withdrawal, denigration, dominance/intimidation; the Profile of Psychological Abuse (MMEA) [68], which measures the dimensions of jealous control, ignore, ridicule traits, and criticize behavior; the Psychological Maltreatment of

Women Inventory (PMWI) [42,69] that assesses the dimensions of dominance/isolation and Emotional/verbal; while other scales, such as the Subtle and Over Psychological Abuse Scale (SOPAS) [46], go beyond assessing distinct dimensions of psychological abuse by simply distinguishing between overt and subtle forms of violence.

1.2. The Scale of Psychological Abuse in Intimate Partner Violence (EAPA-P)

These are complemented by the Scale of Psychological Abuse in Intimate Partner Violence (EAPA-P) [70] which, based on the taxonomy developed by Rodriguez-Carballeira and colleagues [71] provides for the measurement of different strategies of psychological violence, from the most obvious to the most subtle, as outlined by Marshall [46]. EAPA-P begins, then, with the consideration that psychological violence, defined as *"continued application of strategies of pressure, control, manipulation and coercion with the purpose of dominating and subjugating the partner"* [70], can be enacted with direct strategies (influence on the emotions, cognitions, and behaviors of the partner) or with indirect strategies (control). This makes it possible to avoid a strict classification based solely on the tactics used by the perpetrator, thus allowing for a broadening of the acts themselves that are evaluated, considering instead the mode of violence acted out.

The validation of the original version of the EAPA-P involved a sample of 101 women with a mean age of 51.29 (SD = 13.04; range = 24–82) living in Spain and recruited through different municipal services that attend to these victims. Of these, 76% stated that they had experienced physical violence, 65% sexual violence, and 100% psychological violence. The 47 source items were formulated based on the taxonomy of psychological abuse strategies by Rodriguez-Carballeira and colleagues [71]. Following total item-scale, subscale, and corrected item-total correlations and exploratory factor analyses, 19 items were selected. A series of confirmatory analyses were conducted on this one, which indicated that the best model was the two-factor model: direct emotional abuse strategies and indirect emotional abuse strategies. The scale showed excellent internal consistency (α = 0.92) and convergent validity with the Subtle and Overt Psychological Abuse Scale [46], the Hospital Anxiety and Depression Scale [72], and the Davidson Trauma Scale [73].

The primary aim of this study is to develop an Italian version of EAPA-P [70] and to assess its psychometric properties. Furthermore, the concurrent validity of the EAPA-P was examined to provide additional information on the validity of this instrument.

Research Question 1: Investigate the psychometric properties of the Italian version of EAPA-P among a group of Italian-speaker women who reported to experience psychological violence

Research Question 2: Investigate how strongly the Italian version of EAPA-P correlates with other factors related to psychological violence

Research Question 3: Investigate the capacity of the Italian version of EAPA-P to discriminate among women who reported to experience psychological violence and who don't.

2. Materials and Methods

2.1. Participants

A convenience sample of 452 participants, was recruited among adult population from Centers Against Domestic Violence as well as by voluntary participation through online recruitment within websites for listening and support for victims of violence. Anonymity and the right to refuse participation were guaranteed. The questionnaire was spread through the Qualtrics platform (Qualtrics.XM https://www.qualtrics.com/ accessed on 1 June 2021), including the requirement to fill in all questions in order not to have missing data. Participants could refuse their consent to fill in the questionnaire and drop out at any time. Inclusion criteria were to be a woman or self-identify as a woman (since the original version of the EAPA-P was validated on a sample of women), to be an Italian native speaker, to be of legal age, to have given their consent to the research and to fill in the entire EAPA-P scale. Three participants decided not to give their consent to participate in the study, and 106 participants did not fill in the entire EAPA-P scale therefore, the final sample comprised 343 participants. Sample characteristics were as follows: mean age was 26.62 years (SD = 6.33; range = 18–65); the sexual orientation was distributed as follows: 1.5% self-identified as asexual, 80.5% self-identified as heterosexual, 11.7% self-identified as bisexual, 1.8% self-identified as homosexual, 2.9% self-identified as pansexual and 1.5% self-identified as queer/other sexual orientation. 78.7% of the final sample referred they had never experienced physical violence from a partner, 18.4% had experienced it, and 2.9% chose not to answer the question; 43.7% did not experience psychological abuse from a partner, 52.2% had experienced it, and 4.1% chose not to answer the question (Table 1).

Table 1. Descriptive Statistics.

		N	M	SD
Age		343	26.62	6.33
				Valid Percent
Sexual Orientation	Asexual			1.5 (N = 5)
	Heterosexual			80.7 (N = 276)
	Bisexual			11.7 (N = 40)
	Homosexual			1.8 (N = 6)
	Pansexual			2.9 (N = 10)
	Queer			1.5 (N = 5)
	Total			100
Experienced Physical Violence?	No			78.7 (N = 270)
	Yes			18.4 (N = 63)
	Did not report			2.9 (N = 10)
	Total			100
Experienced Psychological Violence?	No			43.7 (N = 150)
	Yes			52.2 (N = 179)
	Did not report			4.1 (N = 14)
	Total			100

Note. M = Mean; SD = Standard Deviation.

This study was conducted in accordance with the ethical standards of the Helsinki Declaration and was approved by the Institutional Review Board of the Department of Psychology of "Sapienza" University of Rome prot. N. 0000866.

2.2. Materials

An ad hoc online questionnaire was designed to collect personal information (i.e., gender, age, sexual orientation, history of physical and/or psychological abuse), and was distributed through different channels, such as Centers Against Domestic Violence and websites for listening and support for victims of violence. The questionnaire included the EAPA-P scale and the measures described in the next sections.

2.2.1. Italian Translation of EAPA-P

Two independent researchers with excellent knowledge of English and psychological vocabulary translated the questionnaire from the English version of EAPA-P into Italian and then agreed on a common version. In this phase, particular care and attention were paid to avoid the presence of colloquial expressions, slang, or unintelligible or ambiguous phrases.

In the second phase, the common version was translated into English (back-translation) by a bilingual person with an extensive knowledge of psychological vocabulary; after correcting some translation inaccuracies, the final Italian version was obtained.

2.2.2. Difficulties in Emotion Regulation Strategies-20 (DERS-20)

The Difficulties in Emotion Regulation Scales-20 [74] provides an assessment of emotional dysregulation across the following subscales: Non Acceptance (i.e., lack of acceptance of the emotional response); Impulse (i.e., difficulty in impulse control when experiencing negative emotions); Goals (i.e., difficulty distracting oneself from the emotion and performing alternative behaviors); Awareness (i.e., lack of emotional self-awareness); and Clarity (i.e., difficulty recognizing the emotion experienced); it is a self-reported questionnaire consisting in 20-items (e.g., "I pay attention to how I feel"), on a 5-point Likert scale, running from "Almost never" (1) to "Almost always" (5) (α = 0.921)

2.2.3. Interpersonal Guilt Rating Scale (IGRS-15)

The Interpersonal Guilt Rating Scales-15s [75] is a measure used for assessing interpersonal guilt. The scale allows for the detection of three constructs: Survivor Guilt (i.e., a painful emotion felt when the person feels they have been more "fortunate" than others and views this as unfair), Self-Hatred (i.e., feeling of being inadequate, wrong, and not deserving of acceptance, love and happiness), and Omnipotence Guilt (which consists in two different sub-factors, the sense of separation/disloyalty and the omnipotent responsibility); interpersonal guilt is assessed through 15-items (e.g., "I feel uncomfortable feeling better off than other people") on a 5-point Likert scale, running from "Not representative at all" (1) to "Completely representative" (5) (α = 0.874).

2.2.4. Revised Conflict Tactic Scale (CTS-2)

The Revised Conflict Tactics Scale [51] is a 78-item measure of Intimate Partner Violence. The scale provides an assessment of both the victimization aspect (39 items) and the perpetration aspect (39 items) of violence. Consistent with the EAPA-P validation aim, only the scale that assesses the victimization aspects (i.e., negotiation, physical violence, psychological violence, physical injury, and sexual violence) have been used. Participants are asked to state how many times a specific situation happened in the previous year (e.g., "My partner threw something at me that could hurt") on an 8-point frequency scale ranging from never to more than 20 times (α = 0.852).

2.2.5. Depression Anxiety Stress Scales (DASS-21)

The Depression Anxiety Stress Scales [76] allows for the detection of three constructs: Depression, Anxiety, Stress. Depression includes dysphoria, hopelessness, devaluing life, lack of interest/involvement, anhedonia, and inertia; Anxiety relates to autonomic nervous system arousal, skeletal muscle effects, situational anxiety, and subjective experience of anxious affects; Stress relates to the presence of nonspecific arousal levels, difficulty relaxing, nervous excitement, irritability, agitation, hyperactivity, and impatience. Answers are assessed through 21 items (e.g., "I found it difficult to relax") on a 4-point Likert scale ranging from "Did not apply to me at all" (0) to "Applied to me very much or most of the time" (3) (α = 0.954).

2.3. Data Analyses

Preliminarily, the CFA was conducted to verify the correspondence between the data obtained and the factorial structure proposed by the authors [70]. Once the values of the goodness of adaptation had been verified, an exploratory factor analysis (EFA) was carried out to identify the factorial structure in our sample. The analyses yielded a two-factor factorial structure. Based on this factorial structure, the items with a main saturation value lower than 0.4 and the presence of secondary saturations that were higher than half of the value of the main saturation [77] were removed. We obtained a 11-item structure on which an additional CFA and EFA were conducted to verify that the structure showed good fit indices and the presence of the original two-factor structure; afterward, reliability analyses were carried out.

To evaluate the concurrent validity of the EAPA-P with the other measures, the correlations between the EAPA-P, the DERS-20, the IGRS-15, the CTS-2, the DASS-21, and their subscales have been conducted. MPlus version 7 [78] was used to conduct the confirmatory factor analysis (CFA), while SPSS (statistical package version 25.0 (IBM, Armonk, NY, USA)) was used for the remaining analyses.

3. Results

3.1. Factorial Analysis

A maximum likelihood confirmatory factor analysis (CFA) was initially conducted to verify the correspondence between the data obtained and the factor structure proposed by the authors [70]. Given that the values of the indices obtained ($\chi2(151) = 785.854$, $p < 0.001$; $\chi2/df = 5.20$; RMSEA = 0.11; SRMR = 0.06; CFI = 0.86; AIC = 11265.57; TLI = 0.85) [79–83] weakly supported the original factor structure, an exploratory factor analysis was performed with maximum likelihood extraction method, and varimax with Kaiser normalization rotation method. Kaiser-Meyer-Olkin measure of sampling adequacy was used to examine the appropriateness of factor analysis: a value of 0.934 was obtained, indicting the appropriateness of the factor analysis. The Bartlett's test of sphericity was significant ($p < 0.001$) meaning that our data set was suitable for data reduction. Based on the EFA factor matrix a two-factor solution was obtained. Some items showed a secondary saturation that was higher than half of the value of the main saturation (i.e., items 3, 6, 8, 9, 10, 13, 16) while item 2 did not saturate in any factor in an acceptable way (>0.40) [77]; therefore, these items were removed to maintain the solution's goodness and a new scale consisting in two subscales and 11 items was obtained (Tables 2 and 3). To verify the model fit measures, a new CFA was conducted. The fit measures were: the TLI and CFI were over the threshold value of 0.90 (TLI = 0.92; CFI = 0.94), the SRMR was good (SRMR = 0.047) and the RMSEA was marginal (RMSEA = 0.097).

Table 2. Exploratory Factor Analysis of EAPA-P (N = 343).

Item	Factor 1 (Direct Strategies)	Factor 2 (Indirect Strategies)
EAPA-P4	**0.813**	0.263
EAPA-P5	**0.755**	0.372
EAPA-P12	**0.742**	0.334
EAPA-P7	**0.730**	0.350
EAPA-P11	**0.685**	0.256
EAPA-P3	0.678	0.402
EAPA-P10	0.653	0.346
EAPA-P6	0.605	0.390
EAPA-P9	0.589	0.589
EAPA-P8	0.579	0.552
EAPA-P16	0.564	0.392
EAPA-P1	**0.534**	0.130
EAPA-P2	0.408	0.224
EAPA-P18	0.321	**0.811**
EAPA-P17	0.340	**0.807**
EAPA-P19	0.280	**0.751**
EAPA-P13	0.483	0.659
EAPA-P14	0.234	**0.568**
EAPA-P15	0.204	**0.560**
Average Variance Extracted	0.511	0.502
Composite Reliability	0.861	0.831
% of total variance explained		57.21

Note: Saturations that meet the inclusion criteria are highlighted in bold.

Table 3. EAPA-P scale, Italian and English version.

Factors	Item
Strategie Dirette di Violenza Psicologica "Direct Strategies"	Il mio/La mia partner ha dato un'interpretazione a modo suo degli eventi che ci hanno colpiti. **"My partner interpreted the things that affected us in his own way"** Il mio/La mia partner ha denigrato le mie iniziative o le mie proposte. **"My partner denigrated my initiatives or proposals."** Il mio/La mia partner mi ha trattato/a con disprezzo. **"My partner treated me with scorn."** Il mio/La mia partner mi ha mostrato affetto solo quando gli era utile. **"My partner was affectionate only when it was in his own interest"** Ho annoiato o infastidito il mio/la mia partner esprimendo i miei sentimenti. **"It bothered my partner when I expressed my feelings"** Il mio/La mia partner mi ha dato la colpa di cose per cui non avevo responsabilità. **"My partner blamed me for things I wasn't responsible for"**
Strategie Indirette di Violenza Psicologica "Indirect Strategies"	Il mio/La mia partner ha controllato i nostri soldi e mi ha impedito di utilizzarli ogni volta che poteva. **"My partner controlled our money and restricted my use of it as much as possible"** Il mio/La mia partner mi ha impedito di lasciare liberamente la casa. **"My partner kept me from freely leaving the house"** Il mio/La mia partner mi ha impedito di stabilire legami con le persone a me vicine. **"My partner kept me from establishing relationships with the people around me"** Il mio/La mia partner mi ha impedito di svolgere attività che mi facevano stare bene o che mi piaceva fare. **"My partner kept me from doing activities I felt like doing"** Il mio/La mia partner ha provato ad allontanarmi dalla mia famiglia. **"My partner tried to keep me away from my family members"**

3.2. Internal Consistency

To assess the internal consistency of our scale, a Cronbach's alpha test was performed. Cronbach's alpha was calculated for the total EAPA-P score and for each of the subscales (i.e., "Direct Psychological Abuse (PA) Strategies" and "Indirect PA Strategies"). The results indicated a high internal consistency, with an α of 0.90. The two subscales yielded an α of 0.88 for Direct PA Strategies, and an α of 0.87 for Indirect PA Strategies.

3.3. Concurrent Validity

The correlations among the EAPA-P scales ranged from 0.600 to 0.953; to examine concurrent validity, correlations among the EAPA-P and the other instruments (CTS-2, IGRS-15, DERS-20, DASS-21) have been conducted and are presented in Table 4.

Results showed that the total EAPA-P scale positively correlates with all forms of partner abuse (as measured by the CTS-2), with subdimensions of guilt (e.g., Self-Hate, as measured by the IGRS-15), with emotional dysregulation (DERS-20), and with symptoms of depression, anxiety, and stress (DASS-21), while negatively correlates with negotiation abilities (Negotiation subscale of CTS-2). The EAPA-P Direct PA Strategies subscale follows the same structure as the total scale. Finally, the EAPA-P Indirect PA Strategies subscale follows the same structure as the previous ones but the Omnipotence Guilt and Survivor Guilt subscales of the IGRS-15, the Non-Acceptance, Goals and Clarity subscales of the DERS-20 do not show significant correlations.

Table 4. Concurrent validity among EAPA-P Total Scale, EAPA-P Direct Strategies, EAPA-P Indirect Strategies, and other instruments.

	EAPAP_Total	EAPAP_Direct	EAPAP_Indirect
CTS_Negotiation	−0.298 **	−0.321 **	−0.173 **
CTS_Psychological Violence	0.684 **	0.671 **	0.521 **
CTS_Physical Violence	0.533 **	0.488 **	0.471 **
CTS_Sexual Coercion	0.543 **	0.506 **	0.464 **
CTS_Injury	0.475 **	0.430 **	0.431 **
IGRS_Omnipotence Guilt	0.119 *	0.144 **	0.038
IGRS_Separation/Disloyalty	0.169 **	0.169 **	0.124 *
IGRS_Self-Hate	0.285 **	0.311 **	0.155 **
IGRS_Survivor Guilt	0.159 **	0.167 **	0.101
DERS_NonAcceptance	0.146 **	0.177 **	0.046
DERS_Goals	0.135 *	0.159 **	0.053
DERS_Impulse	0.216 **	0.221 **	0.145 **
DERS_Clarity	0.195 **	0.232 **	0.070
DERS_Awareness	0.231 **	0.213 **	0.201 **
DASS_Depression	0.261 **	0.283 **	0.147 **
DASS_Anxiety	0.290 **	0.292 **	0.207 **
DASS_Stress	0.255 **	0.278 **	0.140 **

Note: ** Correlation is significant at the 0.01 level (2-tailed). * Correlation is significant at the 0.05 level (2-tailed).

3.4. Differences among Groups

A Student's t-test was conducted to compare the group of women who reported experiencing psychological violence (N = 179), those reporting not experiencing it (N = 150), the third group consisting of women who preferred not to report their experience (N = 14) was not considered due to its size. Statistically significant differences emerged between the group who reported having experienced violence and the group who reported not having experienced violence both on the entire EAPA-P scale and on both subscales; in all cases the group who reported having experienced violence showed higher scores on the various scales (Table 5). Cohen's d was used to interpret the effect size, which was large for the total scale and for the direct strategies subscale, while medium for the indirect strategies subscale [84].

Table 5. Comparison between groups on EAPA-P scale and subscales (*t*-test).

	Independent Sample Test							
	t	df	Sig.	d	Multiple Comparisons	Mean Difference	M	SE
EAPA-P_Total	7.274	327	0.000 **	0.805	E vs. nE	4.75	16.49	6.35
EAPA-P_Direct	7.609	327	0.000 **	0.842	E vs. nE	3.58	10.69	4.60
EAPA-P_Indirect	4.525	327	0.000 **	0.501	E vs. nE	1.17	5.80	2.41

Note. ** $p < 0.01$. E = Experienced Psychological Violence; nE = non-Experienced Psychological Violence. M = Mean; SE = Standard Error.

4. Discussion

This study aimed to investigate whether the Italian translation of the EAPA-P scale [70] could be an appropriate instrument to evaluate the presence of psychological abuse strategies in intimate partner relationships among women. Results showed a two-factor solution, like the original Spanish version. Some items (2, 3, 6, 8, 9, 10, 13, 16) showed a secondary saturation greater than half of the main saturation and were therefore removed. Analysis of these items showed that the content was too generic (e.g., item 2, "My partner insisted that in our relationship we should be above the pain and discomfort that each of us could feel") or too extreme (e.g., item 13, "My partner controlled everything I did") and at the same time, a different translation would not have corresponded to the original version. Despite the elimination of these items based on statistical criteria, the content analysis of the factorial structure suggested a retention of the original scale meaning. Exploratory and confirmatory analyses conducted to verify the new 11-item structure showed excellent internal validity and acceptable fit measures.

The correlations of the scale and respective subscales with the psychological constructs selected to assess convergent (CTS-2 except for the Negotiation subscale, IGRS-15, DERS-20, DASS-21) and divergent (Negotiation subscale of CTS-2) validity are in line with the authors' initial hypotheses. Relationships between indirect strategies of psychological violence (measured by EAPA-P), omnipotent and survivor guilt (measured by IGRS-15), non-acceptance of one's emotions, clarity of feeling, and ability to act goal-directed behaviors when upset (measured by DERS-20) did not show significant correlations. Although these constructs are not directly linked among them, we hypothesize that these are all factors most related to more explicit forms of violence.

Comparison between the group of women who reported experiencing psychological violence and the group of women who reported not experiencing it, showed significant differences in both the total scale and the two subscales, with higher values of psychological violence in the first group. This suggests that the EAPA-P, in addition to its acceptable psychometric properties, can correctly discriminate the presence of psychological abuse in the intimate partner relationship.

With respect to the validation of a scale developed in other countries, in this case Spain, there may be a cultural effect on IPV and psychological violence. Overall, studies within the European context have shown that one of the main cultural factors affecting victimization is the gender equality index (GEI). Specifically, women living in low/medium GEI countries are less likely to experience IPV than in high GEI countries. This counterintuitive association is known as the "Nordic paradox" [85], as Northern European countries are those with higher GEIs. This result can be explained by the fact that women living in countries with higher GEI are more able to recognize their exposure to IPV, thus increasing the possibility of detecting episodes of violence. Italy and Spain are neighboring Western European nations and this may explain why in addition to showing similar prevalence of IPV, they also show similar cultures, languages, and social identities [9,85]. Specifically, a study that compared adolescents with respect to psychological violence in Italy and Spain showed that the only descriptive differences between the two countries concerned power imbalance and social support, where the former emerged as higher and the latter lower in Italy, compared to Spain. However, no significant moderation related to the reference country was found, supporting a generalization of the results for the two samples [86].

Despite the importance of developing validated instruments for violence assessment, this study has some limitations. From a conceptual perspective, methodological progress toward defining and operationalizing psychological abuse is needed [35] in order to differentiate between frequencies and severity of the items: as suggested by Dokkedahl [33], items of psychological aggression are often together with items assessing controlling behaviors. The Italian version was obtained from the English version of EAPA-P, which was not the original scale language as done in previous research [87] following the guidelines for translation [88] to reduce the possible translation issues.

Moreover, it should be noted that double translation brings with it difficulties and risks in preserving the original meaning, although double-blind back-translation procedures reduce the possibility of errors, but do not void it. Finally, these assessment instruments are often developed and validated among female populations, despite there are no gender differences in the prevalence of psychological violence [33,89–93]. However, it is important to note that no agreement with respect to this trend appears in the literature. In fact, several studies have found a female [94–97] or male [98,99] prevalence in the perpetration of psychological violence. Given this, the possibility that there are differences with respect to the manner and meaning of violence acted out by the two genders should be considered [100].

For example, men would appear to experience more verbal forms of psychological violence, while women would appear to be more likely to experience controlling behaviors [89].

5. Conclusions

Despite all the limitations, however, this study provides a reliable and validated version of a useful instrument for understanding the assessment of psychological abuse in a female sample and could be broadening used in different research, such as investigate the relationship from psychological abuse and the possible effects on victims' health. To the best of our knowledge, this is the first study in Italy aiming at the validation of an instrument of psychological violence.

The psychometric properties of the EAPA-P suggest that it can be used as an assessing instrument to evaluate the presence of controlling behaviors acted by a partner in female IPV-victims population. However, future studies should broaden the research and the validation also to male and transgender population, moreover, tools such as EAPA-P could be used to investigate the prevalence of psychological abuse phenomenon in different relationship patterns. In fact, psychological violence strategies may differ depending on whether the abusive partner self-identifies as a man or a woman; likewise the frequency and severity of abuse events may change according to the gender of the victim [101–103]. Similarly, future studies could assess the mental health consequences for victims of psychological partner violence, depending on whether it is perpetrated against men, against women, and within different relationship patterns [104,105].

EAPA-P has several clinical implications: firstly, it helps identify forms of psychological violence before they can escalate into other forms of violence; if health professionals can identify violence at its earliest stages, the long-term effects on a woman's health can be minimized [17]. Secondly, the EAPA-P allows us to understand the different psychological violence strategies engaged in by the partner: understanding the mechanisms of violence used can be helpful for structuring increasingly effective support interventions. Psychological violence and its consequences on the population are increasingly getting attention both in research and in crime prevention and reduction of secondary victimization; having validated assessment instruments that can provide data on these phenomena can help authorities and institutions in creating support programs designed for specific communities. Finally, although Italy and Spain would seem to be similar countries and with the same risk factors influencing the possibility of suffering of psychological violence, further studies are needed to understand what differentiates, at a socio-demographic level, women who experienced psychological aggression and women who didn't, and subsequently to compare the two countries.

Author Contributions: Conceptualization, G.L. and C.C.; methodology, G.L.; software, G.L.; validation, G.L., C.C. and B.B.; formal analysis, G.L.; data curation, G.L.; writing—original draft preparation, G.L. and C.C.; writing—review and editing, B.B. and J.B.; supervision, A.M.G.; project administration, G.L. All authors have read and agreed to the published version of the manuscript.

Funding: This research received no external funding.

Institutional Review Board Statement: This study was conducted in accordance with the ethical standards of the Helsinki Declaration and was approved from the Institutional Review Board of the Department of Psychology of "Sapienza" University of Rome prot. N. 0000866.

Informed Consent Statement: Informed consent was obtained from all subjects involved in the study.

Data Availability Statement: The data presented in this study are available on request from the corresponding author. The data are not publicly available due to privacy reason.

Conflicts of Interest: The authors declare no conflict of interest.

References

1. Hall, J.E.; Walters, M.L.; Basile, K.C. Intimate Partner Violence Perpetration by Court-Ordered Men. *J. Interpers. Violence* **2012**, *27*, 1374–1395. [CrossRef]
2. Bair-Merritt, M.H. Intimate Partner Violence. *Pediatr. Rev.* **2010**, *31*, 145–150. [CrossRef]
3. Garcia-Linares, M.I.; Pico-Alfonso, M.A.; Sanchez-Lorente, S.; Savall-Rodriguez, F.; Celda-Navarro, N.; Blasco-Ros, C.; Martinez, M. Assessing Physical, Sexual, and Psychological Violence Perpetrated by Intimate Male Partners toward Women: A Spanish Cross-Sectional Study. *Violence Vict.* **2005**, *20*, 99–123. [CrossRef]
4. WHO. *Violence against Women: Prevalence Estimates, 2018*; World Report on Violence and Health; WHO: Geneva, Switzerland, 2021; pp. 1–112.
5. Elghossain, T.; Bott, S.; Akik, C.; Obermeyer, C.M. Prevalence of intimate partner violence against women in the Arab world: A systematic review. *BMC Int. Health Hum. Rights* **2019**, *19*, 29. [CrossRef]
6. Iqbal, M.; Fatmi, Z. Prevalence of Emotional and Physical Intimate Partner Violence among Married Women in Pakistan. *J. Interpers. Violence* **2021**, *36*, NP4998–NP5013. [CrossRef]
7. Sanz-Barbero, B.; López Pereira, P.; Barrio, G.; Vives-Cases, C. Intimate partner violence against young women: Prevalence and associated factors in Europe. *J. Epidemiol. Community Health* **2018**, *72*, 611–616. [CrossRef]
8. Permanyer, I.; Gomez-Casillas, A. Is the 'Nordic Paradox' an illusion? Measuring intimate partner violence against women in Europe. *Int. J. Public Health* **2020**, *65*, 1169–1179. [CrossRef]
9. Martín-Fernández, M.; Gracia, E.; Lila, M. Psychological intimate partner violence against women in the European Union: A cross-national invariance study. *BMC Public Health* **2019**, *19*, 1739. [CrossRef]
10. Lausi, G.; Pizzo, A.; Cricenti, C.; Baldi, M.; Desiderio, R.; Giannini, A.M.; Mari, E. Intimate partner violence during the covid-19 pandemic: A review of the phenomenon from victims' and help professionals' perspectives. *Int. J. Environ. Res. Public Health* **2021**, *18*, 6204. [CrossRef]
11. Garcia-Moreno, C.; Jansen, H.A.; Ellsberg, M.; Heise, L.; Watts, C.H. Prevalence of intimate partner violence: Findings from the WHO multi-country study on women's health and domestic violence. *Lancet* **2006**, *368*, 1260–1269. [CrossRef]
12. Barchielli, B.; Baldi, M.; Paoli, E.; Roma, P.; Ferracuti, S.; Napoli, C.; Giannini, A.M.; Lausi, G. When "Stay at Home" Can Be Dangerous: Data on Domestic Violence in Italy during COVID-19 Lockdown. *Int. J. Environ. Res. Public Health* **2021**, *18*, 8948. [CrossRef]
13. Maldonado, A.I.; Farzan-Kashani, J.; Sun, S.; Pitts, S.C.; Lorenzo, J.M.; Barry, R.A.; Murphy, C.M. Psychometric Properties and Factor Analysis of a Short Form of the Multidimensional Measure of Emotional Abuse. *J. Interpers. Violence* **2020**, 0886260520957668. [CrossRef]
14. Murphy, C.; O'Leary, K.D. Psychological aggression predicts physical aggression in early marriage. *J. Consult. Clin. Psychol.* **1989**, *57*, 579. [CrossRef]
15. Salis, K.L.; Salwen, J.; O'Leary, K.D. The Predictive Utility of Psychological Aggression for Intimate Partner Violence. *Partn. Abus.* **2014**, *5*, 83–97. [CrossRef]
16. Sullivan, T.P.; McPartland, T.S.; Armeli, S.; Jaquier, V.; Tennen, H. Is it the exception or the rule? Daily co-occurrence of physical, sexual, and psychological partner violence in a 90-day study of substance-using, community women. *Psychol. Violence* **2012**, *2*, 154–164. [CrossRef]
17. Domenech del Rio, I.; Sirvent Garcia del Valle, E. The Consequences of Intimate Partner Violence on Health: A Further Disaggregation of Psychological Violence—Evidence from Spain. *Violence Women* **2017**, *23*, 1771–1789. [CrossRef]
18. Aizpurua, E.; Copp, J.; Ricarte, J.J.; Vázquez, D. Controlling Behaviors and Intimate Partner Violence among Women in Spain: An Examination of Individual, Partner, and Relationship Risk Factors for Physical and Psychological Abuse. *J. Interpers. Violence* **2021**, *36*, 231–254. [CrossRef]
19. Yoshihama, M.; Horrocks, J.; Kamano, S. The Role of Emotional Abuse in Intimate Partner Violence and Health among Women in Yokohama, Japan. *Am. J. Public Health* **2009**, *99*, 647–653. [CrossRef]
20. Leisring, P.A. Physical and Emotional Abuse in Romantic Relationships. *J. Interpers. Violence* **2013**, *28*, 1437–1454. [CrossRef]
21. Follingstad, D.R.; Rutledge, L.L.; Berg, B.J.; Hause, E.S.; Polek, D.S. The role of emotional abuse in physically abusive relationships. *J. Fam. Violence* **1990**, *5*, 107–120. Available online: http://link.springer.com/10.1007/BF00978514 (accessed on 18 June 2021). [CrossRef]
22. Estefan, L.F.; Coulter, M.L.; VandeWeerd, C. Depression in Women Who Have Left Violent Relationships. *Violence Women* **2016**, *22*, 1397–1413. [CrossRef] [PubMed]
23. Reed, G.L.; Enright, R.D. The effects of forgiveness therapy on depression, anxiety, and posttraumatic stress for women after spousal emotional abuse. *J. Consult. Clin. Psychol.* **2006**, *74*, 920–929. [CrossRef]
24. Webb, M.; Heisler, D.; Call, S.; Chickering, S.A.; Colburn, T.A. Shame, guilt, symptoms of depression, and reported history of psychological maltreatment. *Child Abus. Negl.* **2007**, *31*, 1143–1153. [CrossRef]
25. Beck, J.G.; McNiff, J.; Clapp, J.D.; Olsen, S.A.; Avery, M.L.; Hagewood, J.H. Exploring Negative Emotion in Women Experiencing Intimate Partner Violence: Shame, Guilt, and PTSD. *Behav. Ther.* **2011**, *42*, 740–750. [CrossRef] [PubMed]
26. Russell, B.; Ublemann, M.R. Women Surviving an Abusive Relationship: Grief and the Process of Change. *J. Couns. Dev.* **1994**, *72*, 362–367. [CrossRef]

27. Segrin, C. Concordance on Negative Emotion in Close Relationships: Transmission of Emotion or Assortative Mating? *J. Soc. Clin. Psychol.* **2004**, *23*, 836–856. [CrossRef]
28. Ghahari, S.; Davoodi, R.; Yekehfallah, M.; Mazloumi Rad, M. Marital Conflict, Cognitive Emotion Regulation, Maladaptive Schema and Sexual Satisfaction in spouse abused and non-abused women in Iran: A comparative study. *Asian J. Psychiatr.* **2018**, *35*, 1–2. [CrossRef]
29. Mechanic, M.B.; Weaver, T.L.; Resick, P.A. Mental Health Consequences of Intimate Partner Abuse. *Violence Women* **2008**, *14*, 634–654. [CrossRef]
30. Pico-Alfonso, M.A. Psychological intimate partner violence: The major predictor of posttraumatic stress disorder in abused women. *Neurosci. Biobehav. Rev.* **2005**, *29*, 181–193. [CrossRef]
31. Começanha, R.; Basto-Pereira, M.; Maia, Â. Clinically speaking, psychological abuse matters. *Compr. Psychiatry* **2017**, *73*, 120–126. [CrossRef]
32. Gentry, J.; Bailey, B.A. Psychological Intimate Partner Violence during Pregnancy and Birth Outcomes: Threat of Violence versus Other Verbal and Emotional Abuse. *Violence Vict.* **2014**, *29*, 383–392. [CrossRef]
33. Dokkedahl, S.; Kok, R.N.; Murphy, S.; Kristensen, T.R.; Bech-Hansen, D.; Elklit, A. The psychological subtype of intimate partner violence and its effect on mental health: Protocol for a systematic review and meta-analysis. *Syst. Rev.* **2019**, *8*, 198. [CrossRef]
34. Ellsberg, M.; Jansen, H.A.; Heise, L.; Watts, C.H.; Garcia-Moreno, C. Intimate partner violence and women's physical and mental health in the WHO multi-country study on women's health and domestic violence: An observational study. *Lancet* **2008**, *371*, 1165–1172. Available online: https://linkinghub.elsevier.com/retrieve/pii/S014067360860522X (accessed on 12 September 2021). [CrossRef]
35. Heise, L.; Pallitto, C.; García-Moreno, C.; Clark, C.J. Measuring psychological abuse by intimate partners: Constructing a cross-cultural indicator for the Sustainable Development Goals. *SSM-Popul. Health* **2019**, *9*, 100377. [CrossRef]
36. Tiwari, A.; Chan, K.; Fong, D.; Leung, W.; Brownridge, D.; Lam, H.; Wong, B.; Lam, C.; Chau, F.; Chan, A.; et al. The impact of psychological abuse by an intimate partner on the mental health of pregnant women. *BJOG Int. J. Obstet. Gynaecol.* **2008**, *115*, 377–384. [CrossRef]
37. Street, A.E.; Arias, I. Psychological Abuse and Posttraumatic Stress Disorder in Battered Women: Examining the Roles of Shame and Guilt. *Violence Vict.* **2001**, *16*, 65–78.
38. Pica, E.; Sheahan, C.L.; Pozzulo, J. Examining Mock Jurors' Perceptions of Intimate Partner Violence Factors. *Partn. Abus.* **2019**, *10*, 391–408. [CrossRef]
39. Jewkes, R. Emotional abuse: A neglected dimension of partner violence. *Lancet* **2010**, *376*, 851–852.
40. Follingstad, D.R. Rethinking current approaches to psychological abuse: Conceptual and methodological issues. *Aggress. Violent Behav.* **2007**, *12*, 439–458. Available online: https://linkinghub.elsevier.com/retrieve/pii/S1359178907000031 (accessed on 25 May 2021). [CrossRef]
41. European Institute for Gender Equality. *Glossary of Definitions of Rape, Femicide and Intimate Partner Violence*; European Institute for Gender Equality: Vilnius, Lithuania, 2017; pp. 1–52.
42. Tolman, R.M. The Development of a Measure of Psychological Maltreatment of Women by Their Male Partners. *Violence Vict.* **1989**, *4*, 159–177. Available online: http://connect.springerpub.com/lookup/doi/10.1891/0886-6708.4.3.159 (accessed on 30 May 2021).
43. O'Leary, K.D. Psychological Abuse: A Variable Deserving Critical Attention in Domestic Violence. *Violence Vict.* **1999**, *14*, 3–23. [CrossRef]
44. Lawrence, E.; Orengo-Aguayo, R.; Langer, A.; Brock, R.L. The Impact and Consequences of Partner Abuse on Partners. *Partn. Abus.* **2012**, *3*, 406–428. [CrossRef]
45. Podaná, Z. Patterns of intimate partner violence against women in Europe: Prevalence and associated risk factors. *J. Epidemiol. Community Health* **2021**, *75*, 772–778. Available online: https://jech.bmj.com/lookup/doi/10.1136/jech-2020-214987 (accessed on 23 September 2021). [CrossRef] [PubMed]
46. Marshall, L.L. Effects of Men's Subtle and Overt Psychological Abuse on Low-Income Women. *Violence Vict.* **1999**, *14*, 69–88. [CrossRef]
47. Marshall, L.L. Physical and Psychological Abuse. In *The Dark Side of Interpersonal Communication*; Cupach, W.R., Spitzberg, B.H., Eds.; Routledge: London, UK, 1994; pp. 281–312.
48. Kishor, S.; Johnson, K. *Profiling Domestic Violence: A Multi-Country Study*; ORC Macro: Calverton, MD, USA, 2004.
49. McClintock, H.F.; Trego, M.L.; Wang, E.M. Controlling Behavior and Lifetime Physical, Sexual, and Emotional Violence in sub-Saharan Africa. *J. Interpers. Violence* **2021**, *36*, 7776–7801. [CrossRef]
50. Rodenburg, F.A.; Fantuzzo, J.W. The measure of wife abuse: Steps toward the development of a comprehensive assessment technique. *J. Fam. Violence* **1993**, *8*, 203–228. [CrossRef]
51. Straus, M.; Hamby, S.L.; Boney-McCoy, S.; Sugarman, D.B. The Revised Conflict Tactics Scales (CTS2). *J. Fam. Issues* **1996**, *17*, 283–316. [CrossRef]
52. Hamby, S.L. The Dominance Scale: Preliminary Psychometric Properties. *Violence Vict.* **1996**, *11*, 199–212. [CrossRef]
53. Shepard, M.F.; Campbell, J.A. The Abusive Behavior Inventory. *J. Interpers. Violence* **1992**, *7*, 291–305. [CrossRef]
54. Hegarty, K.; Sheehan, M.; Schonfeld, C. A multidimensional definition of partner abuse: Development and preliminary validation of the composite abuse scale. *J. Fam. Violence* **1999**, *14*, 399–415. [CrossRef]

55. Hegarty, K.; Bush, R.; Sheehan, M. The composite abuse scale: Further development and assessment of reliability and validity of a multidimensional partner abuse measure in clinical settings. *Violence Vict.* **2005**, *20*, 529–547. [CrossRef] [PubMed]
56. Sullivan, C.M.; Bybee, D.I. Reducing violence using community-based advocacy for women with abusive partners. *J. Consult. Clin. Psychol.* **1999**, *67*, 43–53. [CrossRef]
57. Attala, J.M.; Hudson, W.W.; McSweeney, M.; Features Submission, H.C. A partial validation of two short-form partner abuse scales. *Women Health* **1994**, *21*, 125–139. [CrossRef]
58. Straus, M.; Hamby, S.L.; Warren, W.L. *The Conflict Tactics Scale Handbook*; Western Psychological Services: Los Angeles, CA, USA, 2003.
59. Foshee, V.A.; Bauman, K.E.; Arriaga, X.B.; Helms, R.W.; Koch, G.G.; Linder, G.F. An evaluation of Safe Dates, an adolescent dating violence prevention program. *Am. J. Public Health* **1998**, *88*, 45–50. [CrossRef] [PubMed]
60. Foshee, V.A.; Fletcher Linder, G.; Bauman, K.E.; Langwick, S.A.; Arriaga, X.B.; Heath, J.L.; McMahon, P.M.; Bangdiwala, S. The Safe Dates Project: Theoretical Basis, Evaluation Design, and Selected Baseline Findings. *Am. J. Prev. Med.* **1996**, *12*, 39–47. [CrossRef]
61. Smith, P.H.; Smith, J.B.; Earp, J.A.L. Beyond the measurement trap: A reconstructed conceptualization and measurement of woman battering. *Psychol. Women Q.* **1999**, *23*, 177–193. [CrossRef]
62. Smith, P.H.; Earp, J.A.; DeVellis, R. Measuring battering: Development of the Women's Experience with Battering (WEB) Scale. *Womens Health* **1995**, *1*, 273–288. [PubMed]
63. Smith, P.H.; Thornton, G.E.; DeVellis, R.; Earp, J.; Coker, A.L. A Population-Based Study of the Prevalence and Distinctiveness of Battering, Physical Assault, and Sexual Assault in Intimate Relationships. *Violence Women* **2002**, *8*, 1208–1232. [CrossRef]
64. Jones, S.; Davidson, W.S.; Bogat, G.A.; Levendosky, A.; von Eye, A. Validation of the Subtle and Overt Psychological Abuse Scale: An Examination of Construct Validity. *Violence Vict.* **2005**, *20*, 407–416. Available online: http://openurl.ingenta.com/content/xref?genre=article&issn=0886-6708&volume=20&issue=4&spage=407 (accessed on 25 May 2021). [CrossRef]
65. Follingstad, D.R.; Dehart, D.D. Defining psychological abuse of husbands toward wives: Contexts, behaviors, and typologies. *J. Interpers. Violence* **2000**, *15*, 891–920. [CrossRef]
66. Murphy, C.; Hoover, S.A.; Taft, C. *The Multidimensional Measure of Emotional Abuse: Factor Structure and Subscale Validity*; Association for Advancement of Behavior Therapy: Toronto, ON, Canada, 1999.
67. Murphy, C.M.; Hoover, S.A. Measuring Emotional Abuse in Dating Relationships as a Multifactorial Construct. *Violence Vict.* **1999**, *14*, 39–53. [CrossRef]
68. Sackett, L.A.; Saunders, D.G. The impact of different forms of psychological abuse on battered women. *Violence Vict.* **1999**, *14*, 105–117. [CrossRef]
69. Tolman, R.M. The Validation of the Psychological Maltreatment of Women Inventory. *Violence Vict.* **1999**, *14*, 25–37. [CrossRef]
70. Porrúa-García, C.; Rodríguez-Carballeira, Á.; Escartín, J.; Gómez-Benito, J.; Almendros, C.; Martín-Peña, J. Desarrollo y validación de la escala de abuso psicológico aplicado en la pareja (EAPA-P). *Psicothema* **2016**, *28*, 214–221.
71. Rodríguez-Carballeira, A.; Porrúa-García, C.; Escartín, J.; Martín-Peña, J.; Almendros, C. Taxonomy and hierarchy of psychological abuse strategies in intimate partner relation-ships. [Taxonomía y jerarquización de las estrategias de abuso psicológico en la violencia de pareja]. *An. Psicol.* **2014**, *30*, 916–926. [CrossRef]
72. López-Roig, S.; Terol, M.C.; Pastor, M.A.; Neipp, M.C.; Massutí, B. Ansiedad y depresión. Validación de la escala HAD en pacientes oncológicos. *Rev. Psicol. Salud* **2000**, *12*, 127–155.
73. Bobes, J.; Calcedo-Barba, A.; García, M.; François, M.; Rico-Villademoros, F.; González, M.P.; Bousoño, M. Evaluación de las propiedades psicométricas de la versión española de cinco cuestionarios para la evaluación del trastorno de estrés postraumático. *Actas Esp. Psiquiatr.* **2000**, *28*, 207–218.
74. Lausi, G.; Quaglieri, A.; Burrai, J.; Mari, E.; Giannini, A.M. Development of the DERS-20 among the Italian population: A study for a short form of the Difficulties in Emotion Regulation Scale. *Mediterr. J. Clin. Psychol.* **2020**, *8*. [CrossRef]
75. Gazzillo, F.; Gorman, B.; De Luca, E.; Faccini, F.; Bush, M.; Silberschatz, G.; Dazzi, N. Preliminary Data about the Validation of a Self-Report for the Assessment of Interpersonal Guilt: The Interpersonal Guilt Rating Scales–15s (IGRS-15s). *Psychodyn. Psychiatry* **2018**, *46*, 23–48. [CrossRef]
76. Lovibond, P.F.; Lovibond, S.H. The structure of negative emotional states: Comparison of the Depression Anxiety Stress Scales (DASS) with the Beck Depression and Anxiety Inventories. *Behav. Res. Ther.* **1995**, *33*, 335–343. [CrossRef]
77. Barbaranelli, C.; D'Olimpio, F. *Analisi Dei Dati con SPSS*; Led Milano: Milan, Italy, 2006; Volume 2.
78. Muthén, B.; Muthén, L. *Mplus*; Chapman and Hall/CRC: London, UK, 2017.
79. Barbaranelli, C.; Ingoglia, S. *I Modelli di Equazioni Strutturali: Temi e Prospettive*; Led Milano: Milan, Italy, 2013.
80. Bentler, P.M.; Bonett, D.G. Significance tests and goodness of fit in the analysis of covariance structures. *Psychol. Bull.* **1980**, *88*, 588–606. [CrossRef]
81. Hu, L.; Bentler, P.M. Fit indices in covariance structure modeling: Sensitivity to underparameterized model misspecification. *Psychol. Methods* **1998**, *3*, 424–453. [CrossRef]
82. Browne, M.W.; Cudeck, R. Alternative Ways of Assessing Model Fit. *Sociol. Methods Res.* **1992**, *21*, 230–258. [CrossRef]
83. Schermelleh-Engel, K.; Moosbrugger, H.; Müller, H. Evaluating the fit of structural equation models: Tests of significance and descriptive goodness-of-fit measures. *Methods Psychol. Res. Online* **2003**, *8*, 23–74.

84. Magnusson, K. Interpreting Cohen's d effect size: An interactive visualization (Version 2.5.1). *R Psychologist* 2021. Available online: https://rpsychologist.com/cohend/ (accessed on 16 November 2021).
85. Gracia, E.; Merlo, J. Intimate partner violence against women and the Nordic paradox. *Soc. Sci. Med.* **2016**, *157*, 27–30. [CrossRef] [PubMed]
86. Menesini, E.; Nocentini, A.; Ortega-Rivera, F.J.; Sanchez, V.; Ortega, R. Reciprocal involvement in adolescent dating aggression: An Italian–Spanish study. *Eur. J. Dev. Psychol.* **2011**, *8*, 437–451. [CrossRef]
87. Nishimori, M.; Moerman, N.; Fukuhara, S.; Van Dam, F.S.A.M.; Muller, M.J.; Hanaoka, K.; Yamada, Y. Translation and validation of the Amsterdam preoperative anxiety and information scale (APAIS) for use in Japan. *Qual. Life Res.* **2002**, *11*, 361–364. [CrossRef]
88. Behling, O.; Law, K.S. *Translating Questionnaires and Other Research Instruments: Problems and Solutions*; Sage: Southend Oaks, CA, USA, 2000; Volume 133.
89. Dim, E.E.; Elabor-Idemudia, P. Prevalence and Predictors of Psychological Violence against Male Victims in Intimate Relationships in Canada. *J. Aggress. Maltreat. Trauma* **2018**, *27*, 846–866. [CrossRef]
90. Black, M.; Basile, K.; Breiding, M.; Smith, S.; Walters, M.; Merrick, M.; Chen, J.; Stevens, M. *National Intimate Partner and Sexual Violence Survey: 2010 Summary Report*; Centers for Disease Control and Prevention (CDC): Atlanta, GA, USA, 2011.
91. Breiding, M.J.; Smith, S.G.; Basile, K.C.; Walters, M.L.; Chen, J.; Merrick, M.T. Prevalence and characteristics of sexual violence, stalking, and intimate partner violence victimization–national intimate partner and sexual violence survey, United States, 2011. *MMWR. Surveill. Summ.* **2014**, *63*, 1–18. Available online: http://www.ncbi.nlm.nih.gov/pubmed/25188037 (accessed on 18 September 2021).
92. Carney, M.M.; Barner, J.R. Prevalence of Partner Abuse: Rates of Emotional Abuse and Control. *Partn. Abus.* **2012**, *3*, 286–335. [CrossRef]
93. Follingstad, D.R.; Edmundson, M. Is Psychological Abuse Reciprocal in Intimate Relationships? Data from a National Sample of American Adults. *J. Fam. Violence* **2010**, *25*, 495–508. [CrossRef]
94. Frieze, I.H. Female Violence against Intimate Partners: An Introduction. *Psychol. Women Q.* **2005**, *29*, 229–237. [CrossRef]
95. Hamby, S. The gender debate about intimate partner violence: Solutions and dead ends. *Psychol. Trauma Theory Res. Pract. Policy* **2009**, *1*, 24–34. [CrossRef]
96. Langhinrichsen-Rohling, J. Controversies Involving Gender and Intimate Partner Violence in the United States. *Sex Roles* **2010**, *62*, 179–193. [CrossRef]
97. McHugh, M.C. Understanding Gender and Intimate Partner Abuse. *Sex Roles* **2005**, *52*, 717–724. [CrossRef]
98. McHugh, M.C.; Rakowski, S.; Swiderski, C. Men's Experience of Psychological Abuse: Conceptualization and Measurement Issues. *Sex Roles* **2013**, *69*, 168–181. [CrossRef]
99. Romito, P.; Beltramini, L.; Escribà-Agüir, V. Intimate Partner Violence and Mental Health among Italian Adolescents. *Violence Women* **2013**, *19*, 89–106. [CrossRef]
100. Dixon, L.; Graham-Kevan, N. Understanding the nature and etiology of intimate partner violence and implications for practice and policy. *Clin. Psychol. Rev.* **2011**, *31*, 1145–1155. [CrossRef]
101. Rogers, M.J.; Follingstad, D. Gender differences in reporting psychological abuse in a national sample. *J. Aggress. Maltreat. Trauma* **2011**, *20*, 471–502. [CrossRef]
102. Caldwell, J.E.; Swan, S.C.; Woodbrown, V.D. Gender differences in intimate partner violence outcomes. *Psychol. Violence* **2012**, *2*, 42. [CrossRef]
103. Chan, K.L. Gender differences in self-reports of intimate partner violence: A review. *Aggress. Violent Behav.* **2011**, *16*, 167–175. [CrossRef]
104. Thureau, S.; Le Blanc-Louvry, I.; Thureau, S.; Gricourt, C.; Proust, B. Conjugal violence: A comparison of violence against men by women and women by men. *J. Forensic Leg. Med.* **2015**, *31*, 42–46. [CrossRef]
105. Coker, A.L.; Davis, K.E.; Arias, I.; Desai, S.; Sanderson, M.; Brandt, H.M.; Smith, P.H. Physical and mental health effects of intimate partner violence for men and women. *Am. J. Prev. Med.* **2002**, *23*, 260–268. [CrossRef]

Article

Factors Related to Women's Psychological Distress during the COVID-19 Pandemic: Evidence from a Two-Wave Longitudinal Study

Maria Di Blasi [1,*], Gaia Albano [1,*], Giulia Bassi [2,3], Elisa Mancinelli [2,3], Cecilia Giordano [1], Claudia Mazzeschi [4], Chiara Pazzagli [4], Silvia Salcuni [2], Gianluca Lo Coco [1], Omar Carlo Gioacchino Gelo [5,6], Gloria Lagetto [5], Maria Francesca Freda [7], Giovanna Esposito [7], Barbara Caci [1], Aluette Merenda [1] and Laura Salerno [1]

[1] Department of Psychology, Educational Science and Human Movement, University of Palermo, 90128 Palermo, Italy; cecilia.giordano@unipa.it (C.G.); gianluca.lococo@unipa.it (G.L.C.); barbara.caci@unipa.it (B.C.); aluette.merenda@unipa.it (A.M.); laura.salerno@unipa.it (L.S.)
[2] Department of Developmental and Social Psychology, University of Padova, 35132 Padova, Italy; giulia.bassi@phd.unipd.it (G.B.); elisa.mancinelli@phd.unipd.it (E.M.); silvia.salcuni@unipd.it (S.S.)
[3] Digital Health Lab, Fondazione Bruno Kessler, 38122 Trento, Italy
[4] Department of Philosophy, Social & Human Sciences and Education, University of Perugia, 06123 Perugia, Italy; claudia.mazzeschi@unipg.it (C.M.); chiara.pazzagli@unipg.it (C.P.)
[5] Department of History, Society and Human Studies, University of Salento, 73100 Lecce, Italy; omar.gelo@unisalento.it (O.C.G.G.); gloria.lagetto@unisalento.it (G.L.)
[6] Faculty of Psychotherapy Science, Sigmund Freud University Vienna, 1020 Vienna, Austria
[7] Department of Humanities, University of Napoli Federico II, 80133 Napoli, Italy; mariafrancesca.freda@unina.it (M.F.F.); giovan.esposito@unina.it (G.E.)
* Correspondence: maria.diblasi@unipa.it (M.D.B.); gaia.albano@unipa.it (G.A.)

Abstract: Background. A growing body of research has highlighted the negative effects of the COVID-19 pandemic on women's mental health. Previous studies showed that women have higher levels of depression, anxiety and PTSD, and worse psychological adjustment than men, which also persisted after the earlier phase of the pandemic. This study aimed to evaluate changes in women's psychological distress during the pandemic and to evaluate the factors that have a more significant impact in predicting women's psychological distress. Methods. This two-wave longitudinal study (T1 = Italian first lockdown, and T2 = second phase, when the restrictive measures were eased) involved 893 women (M_{age} = 36.45, SD = 14.48). Participants provided demographic and health data as well as measures of psychological distress, emotion regulation processes, and ability to tolerate uncertainty. Results. No significant changes were found in women's psychological distress between T1 and T2, i.e., during and after the first lockdown. Lower social stability status and higher maladaptive emotional coping predicted high psychological distress. Conclusions. Results showed that modifiable psychological variables play a central role in predicting distress and indicated that emotion regulation interventions might be helpful in increasing psychological resilience and mitigating the adverse impacts of the COVID-19 pandemic within the female population.

Keywords: women; COVID-19; distress; principal component analysis; emotion regulation; social stability status; intolerance of uncertainly

1. Introduction

The worldwide spread of COVID-19 and subsequent mitigation measures have caused a significant increase in mental health problems in many countries.

In addition to the primary threat of infection, social distancing measures to combat the spread of the virus have also had negative psychological, social, and economic consequences on the general population [1,2]. Relevant reviews of the consequences of the COVID-19 pandemic on mental health have evidenced increased levels of stress, anxiety and depression, as well as an increase in suicidal ideation across several countries [3–5]. Italy is one of the European countries that have been most dramatically affected by COVID-19. From 9 March 2020 until the 4th of May, the Italian government implemented extraordinary measures to limit the viral transmission, which severely restricted movement of individuals across the whole nation and imposed severe social distancing restrictions. Later, during the second phase, although a large number of preventive and protective measures were still adopted, the mass quarantine was lifted, and restrictive measures were eased. Previous studies on the Italian population showed that, as in the rest of the world, there were high levels of psychological distress and negative mental health effects as a result of the current health emergency [6–8]. Several risk factors, including job loss and economic hardship, reduced sources of social support, increases in familiar disorders and violence, have been linked to worsening levels of mental health during the COVID-19 pandemic [9–11]. Moreover, a growing body of research has also evidenced a more negative mental health impact of the COVID-19 pandemic within specific, vulnerable groups such as women, the young, people with lower educational levels, lower-income, or pre-existing mental health conditions [12–15]. Previous studies on predictors of mental health during COVID-19 evidenced that women had the highest prevalence of mental health problems during the first period of the pandemic [16,17].

In line with these research findings, this study aimed to examine the effects of the pandemic on women's mental health, in order to generate mitigating action that might prevent/alleviate the psychological consequences of the pandemic on women.

Significant gendered pandemic effects may have a negative impact on women's health globally. For example, a greater rate of unemployment among women compared to men during the outbreak has had a detrimental effect on their work and economic opportunities, and increased the pressure to take on caring roles within families as schools and elderly care facilities close [18,19]. Although mortality rates have been twice as high for men as for women [20], the COVID-19 pandemic has affected women's mental health more than men. Several studies highlighted the fact that the increase in women's distress is, in part, due to exacerbated domestic duties, including childcare, linked to working from home and school closures [12,21–23]. This is particularly relevant in the Italian context, where the COVID-19 pandemic has increased the focus on social and cultural inequalities concerning gender, which place Italian women at a greater disadvantage than women from other European countries [18]. Some cross-sectional and longitudinal studies confirmed the negative effects of the COVID-19 pandemic on women's mental health. In a recent study on the general population in Spain, Ausin et al. [12] found significant gender-related differences in the psychological impact of COVID-19, evidencing that women displayed higher levels of depression, anxiety and PTSD, more feelings of loneliness, and less spiritual well-being when compared to men. Similarly, del Río-Casanova et al. [24] found that compared to men, women showed worse psychological adjustment, characterized by a wide range of symptomatology such as anxiety, depression, stress, and posttraumatic symptoms (ranging from mild to moderate). Moreover, a longitudinal study on the trajectories of anxiety and depression over the 20 weeks following the lockdown in England [13] found that although most individuals experienced improvements in mental health when lockdown easing measures were introduced, some vulnerable groups such as women, younger adults, and individuals with lower educational levels showed higher levels of anxiety and depression at the start of lockdown, which decreased but persisted after the earlier phases of confinement.

Although several variables have demonstrated a negative impact on mental health in the general population, little is known about which factors had a greater impact in predicting women's psychological distress during the pandemic. Previous studies [24–26] have examined gender differences in psychological distress after the COVID-19 pandemic, and reported several important factors that were associated with a higher level of mental health problems. In a study conducted in China, Yan et al. [25] found that among female participants, risk factors of distress included poorer health, worse local pandemic status, greater desire for knowledge about COVID-19, the problem of diseases during the pandemic, and an inability to work/study. Conversely, calmness of mood compared with the pre-pandemic period and frequent contact with colleagues were found to act as protective factors against psychological distress. Another recent study [26] found that the caregiving burden, domestic violence, and fear of COVID-19 were independently associated with psychological distress among young women, who presented higher suicide rates during the COVID-19 pandemic.

However, although recent findings shed light on relevant determinants of women's distress during the COVID-19 pandemic, previous studies are limited by their cross-sectional design, emphasizing the need for further longitudinal studies.

Among the psychological factors associated with mental health problems, the way people cope with stressful and unpredictable events was shown to play a crucial role in reducing or heightening psychological distress during the current pandemic [27,28]. For instance, as demonstrated by Parra-Rizo and Sanchìs-Soler (2021) [29], regular physical activity maintains and enhances physical and psychological functioning, facilitating functional independence as well as the absence of diseases in older women. Relevant previous studies have evidenced how the association between emotional regulation strategies and intolerance of incertitude highlighted the negative effects of uncertainty on affect [30,31]. Specifically, a recent study reporting findings from an online survey during initial COVID-19 lockdowns in the United States [32] suggested that the intolerance of uncertainty may impact mental health by reducing the use of adaptive emotion regulation and implementing maladaptive ones. On the other hand, social support and cognitive reappraisal seem to represent protective factors for mental health [7], jointly with perceived coping efficacy, trust in institutional responses to the COVID-19 emergency, perceived house size, and media exposure to the COVID-19 outbreak as citizens' positive and negative mental health predictors [33].

The Present Study

Based on previous studies which showed that women had the highest prevalence of mental health problems during the first period of the COVID-19 pandemic [16,17], the aims of the present study were twofold: (a) to evaluate changes in women's psychological distress between the first (T1) and the second phases (T2) of the lockdown in Italy (April–May 2020), and (b) to evaluate the role of certain relevant demographic, health, and psychological factors in predicting women's psychological distress. Thus, the following hypotheses were tested:

Hypothesis 1 (H1). *Consistently with previous studies, suggesting that women's levels of anxiety and depression persisted after the earlier phase of the pandemic [13], we predicted no significant improvement in psychological distress from T1 to T2.*

Hypothesis 2 (H2). *We expected that psychological distress at T2 would be predicted by factors such as demographic and health profile, COVID-19-related factors, intolerance of uncertainty, and emotion regulation strategies.*

2. Materials and Methods

2.1. Participants and Procedure

Eligible participants were included if they were aged 18 or over, spoke Italian as their first language, and if they were able to access an electronic device (e.g., mobile phone, computer, laptop, or tablet) connected to the Internet. Data were collected during a period of national lockdown, in two different waves, between the 7th and 24th April 2020 (during the first phase of the COVID-19 outbreak) and between the 18th and 31st May 2020 (during the second phase when the restrictive measures were eased). Participants completed a baseline online assessment on the Google Form web platform (https://docs.google.com/

forms/u/0/). The study was conducted according to the guidelines of the Declaration of Helsinki, and approved by the Ethics Committee of the University of Palermo.

The study included a total of 893 women (mean age = 36.45; SD = 14.48). At Time 1, data were collected from 2915 women, as part of a larger study on the psychological consequences of the COVID-19 pandemic. Of this initial sample, 490 (16.8%) were not available to complete the survey at T2. Of the remaining 2425 women, 893 (36.8%) participated in the second wave (Time 2). Only women who provided both T1 and T2 data were included in the present study. Participants' demographic information is reported in Table 1.

Table 1. Demographics and health-related data.

	Sample n = 893
Age, M (SD)	36.45 (14.48)
Educational level, n (%)	
13 years of schooling	303 (34.0)
Degree/post-graduate	590 (66.0)
Employment status, n (%)	
Unemployed	401 (44.9)
Employed (part-time/full-time)	492 (55.1)
Pathologies in the previous year, n (%) yes	66 (7.4)
Diagnosed with a disability, n (%) yes	17 (1.9)
Own diagnosis of COVID-19, n (%) yes	
COVID-19 among relatives, n (%) yes	213 (23.9)

2.2. Measures

Participants completed an online survey consisting of the following measures:

Demographic and health surveys were used at T1 to collect information on the age, level of education, occupation (0 = unemployed, 1 = employed), presence of pathologies in the previous year (e.g., respiratory, cardiac, chronic; 0 = no, 1 = yes), presence of disabilities (0 = no, 1 = yes), evaluation of individual's general health conditions (measured on a 5-point Likert-type scale from 1 "excellent" to 5 "deficient"), and previous COVID-19 diagnosis (0 = no, 1 = yes), or COVID-19 diagnosis among parents/family (0 = no, 1 = yes).

The Depression, Anxiety and Stress Scale (DASS-21) [34,35] is a 21-item self-report scale designed to measure the emotional states of depression, anxiety and stress both at T1 and T2. Participants were asked to indicate the presence of any symptoms over the previous week. Each item is scored from 0 "did not apply to me at all" to 3 "applied to me very much or most of the time". The higher the score, the higher the levels of depression, anxiety, and stress. The DASS-21 showed good to excellent internal consistency in this study (T1 Cronbach's alpha = 0.886, 0.868, and 0.914, for depression, anxiety, and stress subscales, respectively. T2 Cronbach's alpha = 0.899, 0.885, and 0.921 for depression, anxiety, and stress subscales, respectively).

The Emotion Regulation Questionnaire (ERQ) [36,37] was used at T1 to measure individuals' tendency to regulate their emotions through two strategies: (1) Cognitive Reappraisal (i.e., attempts to reinterpret an emotion-eliciting situation in a way that alters its meaning and changes its emotional impact; six items, e.g., "When I want to feel less negative emotions, I change the way I'm thinking about the situation"), and (2) Expressive Suppression (i.e., attempts to reduce or inhibit ingoing emotion-expressive behavior; four items, e.g., "I control my emotions by not expressing them"). Respondents answered each item on a 7-point Likert-type scale, ranging from 1 "strongly disagree" to 7 "strongly agree". The higher the score, the greater the use of that regulation strategy. Cronbach's alpha was 0.886 for the Cognitive Reappraisal subscale, and 0.691 (mean inter-item correlation = 0.357) for the Expressive Suppression subscale.

The Intolerance of Uncertainty Scale-12 (IUS) [38,39] is a 12-item self-report questionnaire (e.g., "When things happen suddenly, I get very upset") used to measure the dispositional inability of an individual to tolerate uncertainty at T1. The IUS-12 covers two domains (i.e., Prospective and Inhibitory) and also provides a total score to evaluate the general intolerance of uncertainty. Respondents are asked to rate the extent to which each statement applies to themselves on a 5-point Likert scale, ranging from 1 "not at all characteristic of me" to 5 "entirely characteristic of me". For the present study, only the total score was used, and it showed good internal consistency (Cronbach's alpha = 0.887).

2.3. Statistical Analyses

As a preliminary step in the data analysis, the normality of continuous variables was checked, and all variables had a normal distribution (Sk: −0.533; 1.566; Ku: −1.001; 2.023). The internal consistency of the scales (Cronbach's α) was computed, and the mean inter-item correlation was examined for the ERQ Expressive Suppression subscale. Mean inter-item correlations between 0.15 and 0.50 indicated adequate internal consistency [40]. Descriptive statistics for continuous (i.e., means and standard deviations) and qualitative variables (i.e., frequencies and percentages) were computed.

To test the first hypothesis of the study, differences in depression, anxiety, and stress (DASS-21) levels between T1 and T2 were tested using a paired samples t-test. Cohen's d effect sizes were also reported.

To test the second hypothesis of the study, data at T1 were summarized by principal component analysis (PCA) with Promax oblique rotation. The applicability of the data for the analysis was verified. The case-to-variable ratio was 81.2 (which exceeds the recommended minimum of 10) [41]. The Kaiser–Meyer–Olkin sampling adequacy measure was 0.587 (Hair et al. [42] suggest accepting a value >0.5), and Bartlett's test of sphericity was significant ($p < 0.001$). The number of factors to retain was determined using visual inspection of the scree plot and an examination of eigenvalues (i.e., factors with eigenvalues greater than 1 were retained). Moreover, multiple regression was computed with factors at T1 as independent variables, and DASS-21 subscales at T2 as dependent variables. Statistical analyses were performed using the Statistical Package for Social Sciences (SPSS), version 22 (IBM Corp., Armonk, NY, USA).

3. Results

3.1. Changes in Psychological Distress between T1 and T2

Table 2 shows descriptive statistics and changes in psychological distress between T1 and T2. At T2 (after the lockdown phase), women reported significantly lower levels of depression, but with a small effect size. No differences between T1 and T2 were found in anxiety and stress levels, nor in the total DASS-21 score.

Table 2. Descriptive statistics and changes in psychological distress between T1 and T2.

	T1 [2]		T2 [3]		T	p	Cohen's d ES [4]
	M	SD	M	SD			
DASS [1]—Depression	8.97	7.01	8.59	7.25	1.975	0.049	0.066
DASS [1]—Anxiety	3.90	4.53	3.75	4.62	1.289	0.198	0.043
DASS [1]—Stress	9.52	5.62	9.42	5.82	0.639	0.523	0.021
DASS [1]—Total Score	20.40	13.80	19.98	14.39	1.170	0.243	0.039

[1] DASS, Depression, Anxiety and Stress Scale; [2] T1, First phase of the COVID-19 outbreak (period of national lockdown, between 7 and 24 April 2020); [3] T2, second phase (when the restrictive measures, between 18 and 31 May 2020); [4] ES, effect size.

3.2. Factors Related to Women's Psychological Distress

As a preliminary step, PCA was used to summarize demographic and health factors, emotion regulation strategies, and intolerance of uncertainty. Both eigenvalues and the visual inspection of the scree plot resulted in the retention of four factors, accounting for 52% of the total variance. Table 3 shows the rotated component matrix with the communalities. The first factor, which explained 16% of the variance, contained three variables and was labeled "Social Stability Status" because it contained demographic data (i.e., age, occupation, and level of education) which are generally related to greater economic security and a more stable social role; the second factor (which explained 14% of the variance) contained three variables and was labeled "Medical Impairment" because it refers to the presence of health diseases unrelated to the COVID-19 pandemic; the third factor (which explains 11% of the variance) contained three variables and was labeled "Maladaptive emotional coping" because it contained data regarding an inability to tolerate uncertainty and maladaptive strategies to regulate emotions; finally, the fourth factor (which explains 10% of the variance) contained two variables and was labeled "Personal contact with COVID-19" because it referred to COVID-19 diagnosis among participants and/or their relatives.

Table 3. Factor loadings and communalities for the rotated matrix.

Variables and Factor Name	Factors				Communalities
	1	2	3	4	
Factor 1: Social Stability Status					
Occupation	0.809				0.666
Level of education	0.651				0.480
Age	0.659				0.512
Factor 2: Medical Impairment					
General health condition		0.734			0.567
Pathologies		0.704			0.497
Disability		0.632			0.442
Factor 3: Maladaptive Emotional Coping					
Intolerance of uncertainty			0.784		0.619
Cognitive Reappraisal			−0.551		0.381
Expressive Suppression			0.678		0.510
Factor 4: Personal contact with COVID-19					
Own COVID-19 diagnosis				0.679	0.482
COVID-19 diagnosis among relatives				0.715	0.524

Subsequently, the contribution of these factors was estimated in order to explain stress, depression, and anxiety levels at T2 (Table 4). A higher social stability status at T1 predicted lower stress, depression, and anxiety levels at T2, whereas higher levels of maladaptive emotional coping at T1 predicted higher stress, depression, and anxiety levels at T2. No significant relationships were found between medical impairment and personal contact with COVID-19 factors and dependent variables. There was no multicollinearity among explanatory variables (maximum variance inflation factor: VIF = 1.033).

Table 4. Regression analyses.

	Adjusted R^2	F	β	p
DV: DASS [1]-stress	0.153	41.198 ***		
Factor 1: Social Stability Status			−0.155	0.000
Factor 2: Medical impairment			0.006	0.855
Factor 3: Maladaptive Emotional Coping			0.341	0.000
Factor 4: Personal contact with COVID-19			−0.048	0.123

Table 4. *Cont.*

	Adjusted R²	F	β	p
DV: DASS¹-depression	0.223	64.940 ***		
Factor 1: Social Stability Status			−0.072	0.016
Factor 2: Medical impairments			0.003	0.933
Factor 3: Maladaptive Emotional Coping			0.460	0.000
Factor 4: Personal contact with COVID-19			−0.039	0.197
DV: DASS¹-anxiety	0.146	39.080 ***		
Factor 1: Social Stability Status			−0.126	0.000
Factor 2: Medical impairments			0.004	0.887
Factor 3: Maladaptive Emotional Coping			0.349	0.000
Factor 4: Personal contact with COVID-19			−0.010	0.750

¹ DASS, Depression, Anxiety and Stress Scale; *** $p < 0.001$.

4. Discussion

The present study surveyed a sample of adult women in two different pandemic waves, between the 7 and 24 April 2020 (T1; during the first phase of the COVID-19 lockdown) and between the 18th and 31st May 2020 (T2; during the second phase of the pandemic, when the restrictive measures were eased) to examine psychosocial variables associated with women's heightened psychological distress. More specifically, we examined changes in depression, anxiety, and stress levels between T1 and T2 and whether demographic, health, and psychological factors predicted women's psychological distress. To the best of our knowledge, this is the first longitudinal study that has examined risk and protective factors of psychological distress in a large-scale national sample of adult women.

In line with our first hypothesis, no significant improvement in the anxiety and stress levels was found from T1 to T2. This finding is in line with certain studies that evidenced a stable pattern of results for psychological distress during the COVID-19 confinement [13], affecting specific at-risk groups such as women [43]. Moreover, Di Blasi et al. [27], in a study with an Italian sample, showed that depression, stress, and anxiety levels represented a "contiguous pattern", which remained stable during the earlier phases of the COVID-19 pandemic. Additionally, previous studies reported that negative impacts of the pandemic on wellbeing have been particularly hard on women, young people, those in lower-income groups, or those who experienced a loss of income [5,44,45].

In the current study, women reported significantly lower levels of depression at T2 (after the lockdown phase), but the effect size was negligible. The slight improvement in our sample seems to corroborate previous studies. For example, Fancourt et al. [13] reported a significant decrease in levels of depression and anxiety over the first 20 weeks following the introduction of a lockdown in England for most individuals, but not for women. Women seem to remain the less recovered and most vulnerable group.

Our second hypothesis was partially supported. More specifically, our results showed that lower social stability status and higher maladaptive emotional coping at T1 predicted higher stress, depression, and anxiety levels at T2. However, no significant relationships were found between "Medical Impairments" and "Personal contact with COVID-19" factors, and dependent variables.

The role of the "Social Stability Status" (i.e., higher age, stable occupation and higher level of education), is consistent with previous studies [5,44,45] and evidenced how the compresence of being young, without a stable paid occupation, and with a low level of education may represent risk factors for psychological distress in women. However, on the other hand, this result indirectly shed light on how the onset of the COVID-19 pandemic has exacerbated existing gender inequalities—namely, in the sphere of economic stability and the gendered divisions of labor—and indicates the need to broaden the focus of research on gender inequalities [46].

Contrary to expectations, no significant relationships were found between "Medical Impairments", "Personal contact with COVID-19" factors, and perceived psychological distress. This result may support the hypothesis that during the early phase of the pandemic, diseases unrelated and/or related to the COVID-19 pandemic might not have significantly affected psychological distress, whereas the socio-demographic and psychological variables have played a central role in predicting a protective role against unexpected circumstances such as COVID-19.

Additionally, from our analyses, higher "Maladaptive Emotional Coping" (i.e., inability to tolerate uncertainty and maladaptive strategies to regulate emotions) is a predictor of higher psychological distress. One of the mechanisms through which suppression and reappraisal have opposite effects on general wellbeing is their association with positive and negative emotions [47,48]. For example, the use of suppression has been associated with decreases in positive impacts and increases in negative impacts [47]. The use of emotion suppression reflects the association between suppression and psychopathology, e.g., symptoms of anxiety and depression [49]. The findings that the inability to tolerate uncertainty and suppression were associated with higher psychological distress is in line with the prediction that unexpected circumstances, such as a pandemic, demand the fostering of skills to regulate negative emotions in tackling distress [50]. Moreover, this result is consistent with those of a recent COVID-19 study [32] which found that an intolerance of uncertainty affects mental health by reducing the use of adaptive emotion regulation.

Furthermore, the present results are significant, considering that a recent study demonstrated that reappraisal interventions could help to increase psychological resilience and alleviate adverse impacts on women, caused by lockdown and self-isolation [51].

Strengths and Limitations

The strengths of this study comprise the use of a longitudinal design and the assessment of modifiable psychological factors, such as emotion regulation. A further strength is the recruitment of individuals from a country (i.e., Italy) which has been most dramatically affected by COVID-19. Nonetheless, findings are limited by potential residual, confounding factors and by the requirement to access a mobile device and possess mobile technology knowledge in order to participate. These criteria might represent an obstacle for participation to those from a less advantageous background and limit the inclusivity of the study. Secondly, the study used a non-random population sample; thus, future studies on more representative samples are needed. Thirdly, the results of this study may have been influenced by Italian social–political–cultural patterns that might limit generalizability to other countries. More specifically, the psychological distress of Italian women during the pandemic may have been exacerbated by social inequalities concerning gender. Previous studies have showed that, in Italy, the percentage of those working in professions with a high risk of infection is higher in women than in men [52]; Italian women have also largely been excluded from participating in decision-making regarding the management of the pandemic and post-pandemic recovery [18]; and since the pandemic began, Italian women have reported increased housework and childcare responsibilities (also due to the inability to access external help as a consequence of the lockdown), and have experienced greater job loss, underemployment and precarious positions in the labor market [18]. Additionally, the high dropout rate is a limitation of this study. This could have been due to the length of the questionnaire and the fact that participants did not receive any compensation for participating in the research. Lastly, the time gap between T1 (during the lockdown phase) and T2 (when the lockdown restrictions were eased) might have been too short to detect a significant change in the individuals' level of psychological distress. Thus, further studies with data collected across multiple time points are needed to confirm our findings.

5. Conclusions

Overall, this study showed that psychological distress in a sample of women remained stable over time, with a trivial decrease in depression from T1 to T2. We also found that a higher social stability status and lower maladaptive emotional coping at T1 predicted lower psychological distress at T2. In this context, the social stability status seems to be associated with a protective role against psychological distress, whereas maladaptive emotional coping can be considered a risk factor for women. Women seem to be at greater risk when coping with negative consequences linked to the COVID-19 outbreak; maladaptive emotion regulation strategies (such as suppression in combination with higher inability to tolerate uncertainty and reduced use of cognitive reappraisal) fostered the vulnerability of the women's group at the time of the first two waves of COVID-19. In summary, the empirical findings of this study provide a new understanding of women's psychological suffering during the novel pandemic, showing how the socio-demographic and psychological variables play a protective role in the face of unexpected circumstances such as COVID-19.

The results of the study have some clinical and social implications. By dealing with the mechanisms behind self-emotional regulation and tolerance of uncertainty, we might help to cope more promptly with all negative consequences due to a worldwide emergency or economic dissatisfaction. Emotion regulation training might strengthen people's resilience towards the pandemic's adverse effects on psychological wellbeing. Specifically, to prevent the chronic manifestations of mental problems, it is necessary to focus psychological preventive and therapeutic interventions on expressing emotions aimed at promoting the use of cognitive reinterpretation of the emotional impact linked to distressing situations. Moreover, policymakers should provide appropriate psychological and social support services to improve women's emotional well-being, aimed at organizing and increasing resources to support individuals and families both during and after any lockdown measure [53]. Finally, further research is needed in order to focus on the gap in gender differences with regard to the impact of outbreaks across several domains. For example, Etheridge and Spantig (2020) [54] found that women's well-being during the pandemic was strongly associated with specific dimensions such as family and caring responsibilities, financial and work situations, and social engagements. Interestingly, this study also found that the gender gap in well-being can be explained by gender differences in social factors. Women reported having more close friends before the pandemic than men, and increased loneliness and well-being declined after the pandemic's onset. This result suggests that lockdown might have impacted women's mental well-being through a strongly adverse and unequal effect of the direct loss of social interaction.

Overall, results from the present study suggest that policymakers should limit the duration of lockdown and social distancing measures, and they should pay particular attention to at-risk groups, mitigating the impact of lockdown on people's social and professional lives as an effective strategy for coping with longer periods.

Author Contributions: M.D.B., G.A. and L.S. designed the study, wrote the protocol, and managed the literature searches. G.A. and L.S. undertook the statistical analysis; M.D.B., G.A. and L.S. wrote the first draft of the manuscript. G.B., E.M., C.G., C.M., C.P., S.S., G.L.C., O.C.G.G., G.L., M.F.F., G.E., B.C. and A.M. critically reviewed the draft of the manuscript, and contributed to the interpretation of results and to the subsequent redrafting of the manuscript. All authors have read and agreed to the published version of the manuscript.

Funding: G.A. was funded by a scholarship from the FFR 2019/2020 fund of the Department of Psychology, Educational Sciences and Human Movement, University of Palermo.

Institutional Review Board Statement: The study was conducted according to the guidelines of the Declaration of Helsinki, and approved by the Ethics Committee of the University of Palermo—Ethics Committee (protocol code n. 3/2020—25 May 2020).

Informed Consent Statement: Informed consent was obtained from all subjects involved in the study.

Data Availability Statement: Data are available from the corresponding authors upon reasonable request.

Conflicts of Interest: The authors declare no conflict of interest.

References

1. Zhang, X.; Cai, H.; Hu, J.; Lian, J.; Gu, J.; Zhang, S.; Ye, C.; Lu, Y.; Jin, C.; Yu, C.; et al. Epidemiological, clinical characteristics of cases of SARS-CoV-2 infection with abnormal imaging findings. *IJID* **2020**, *94*, 81–87. [CrossRef]
2. Nicola, M.; Alsafi, Z.; Sohrabi, C.; Kerwan, A.; Al-Jabir, A.; Iosifidis, C.; Agha, M.; Agha, R. The socio-economic implications of the coronavirus pandemic (COVID-19): A review. *Int. J. Surg.* **2020**, *78*, 185–193. [CrossRef]
3. Brown, E.; Gray, R.; Lo Monaco, S.; O'Donoghue, B.; Nelson, B.; Thompson, A.; Francey, S.; McGorry, P. The potential impact of COVID-19 on psychosis: A rapid review of contemporary epidemic and pandemic research. *Schizophr. Res.* **2020**, *222*, 79–87. [CrossRef]
4. Salari, N.; Hosseinian-Far, A.; Jalali, R.; Vaisi-Raygani, A.; Rasoulpoor, S.; Mohammadi, M.; Rasoulpoor, S.; Khaledi-Paveh, B. Prevalence of stress, anxiety, depression among the general population during the COVID-19 pandemic: A systematic review and meta-analysis. *Glob. Health* **2020**, *16*, 1–11. [CrossRef] [PubMed]
5. Xiong, J.; Lipsitz, O.; Nasri, F.; Lui, L.M.; Gill, H.; Phan, L.; Chen-Li, D.; Iacobucci, M.; Ho, R.; Majeed, A.; et al. Impact of COVID-19 pandemic on mental health in the general population: A systematic review. *J. Affect. Disord.* **2020**, *277*, 55–64. [CrossRef] [PubMed]
6. Ceccato, I.; Palumbo, R.; Di Crosta, A.; Marchetti, D.; La Malva, P.; Maiella, R.; Marin, A.; Mammarella, N.; Verrocchio, M.C.; Di Domenico, A. "What's next?" Individual differences in expected repercussions of the COVID-19 pandemic. *Pers. Individ. Differ.* **2021**, *174*, 106892. [CrossRef]
7. Preti, E.; Pierro, R.D.; Perego, G.; Bottini, M.; Casini, E.; Ierardi, E.; Madeddu, F.; Mazzetti, M.; Riva Crugnola, C.; Taranto, P.; et al. Short-term psychological consequences of the COVID-19 pandemic: Results of the first wave of an ecological daily study in the Italian population. *Psychiatry Res.* **2021**, *305*, 114206. [CrossRef]
8. Roma, P.; Monaro, M.; Colasanti, M.; Ricci, E.; Biondi, S.; Di Domenico, A.; Verrocchio, M.C.; Napoli, C.; Ferracuti, S.; Mazza, C.A. 2-Month Follow-Up Study of Psychological Distress among Italian People during the COVID-19 Lockdown. *Int. J. Environ. Res. Public Health* **2020**, *17*, 8180. [CrossRef]
9. Merenda, A.; Garro, M.; Schirinzi, M. The Invisible Pandemic: Domestic Violence and Health and Welfare Services in Italy and in the United Kingdom during COVID-19. *Int. J. Humanit Soc. Sci. Educ.* **2021**, *8*, 11–20. [CrossRef]
10. Rodríguez-Fernández, P.; González-Santos, J.; Santamaría-Peláez, M.; Soto-Cámara, R.; Sánchez-González, E.; González-Bernal, J.J. Psychological Effects of Home Confinement and Social Distancing Derived from COVID-19 in the General Population—A Systematic Review. *Int. J. Environ. Res. Public Health* **2021**, *18*, 6528. [CrossRef]
11. Wilson, J.M.; Lee, J.; Fitzgerald, H.N.; Oosterhoff, B.; Sevi, B.; Shook, N.J. Job insecurity and financial concern during the COVID-19 pandemic are associated with worse mental health. *J. Occup. Environ. Med.* **2020**, *62*, 686–691. [CrossRef] [PubMed]
12. Ausín, B.; González-Sanguino, C.; Castellanos, M.Á.; Muñoz, M. Gender-related differences in the psycho-logical impact of confinement as a consequence of COVID-19 in Spain. *J. Gend. Stud.* **2021**, *30*, 29–38. [CrossRef]
13. Fancourt, D.; Steptoe, A.; Bu, F. Trajectories of anxiety and depressive symptoms during enforced isolation due to COVID-19 in England: A longitudinal observational study. *Lancet Psychiatry.* **2021**, *8*, 141–149. [CrossRef]
14. Pieh, C.; Budimir, S.; Probst, T. The effect of age, gender, income, work, and physical activity on mental health during coronavirus disease (COVID-19) lockdown in Austria. *J. Psychosom. Res.* **2020**, *136*, 110186. [CrossRef] [PubMed]
15. Kwong, A.S.F.; Pearson, R.M.; Adams, M.J.; Northstone, K.; Tilling, K.; Smith, D.; Fawns-Ritchie, C.; Bould, H.; Warne, N.; Zammit, S.; et al. Mental health before and during the COVID-19 pandemic in two longitudinal UK population cohorts. *Br. J. Psychiatry* **2021**, *218*, 1–10. [CrossRef] [PubMed]
16. Pierce, M.; Hope, H.; Ford, T.; Hatch, S.; Hotopf, M.; John, A.; Kontopantelis, E.; Webb, R.; Wessely, S.; McManus, S.; et al. Mental health before and during the COVID-19 pandemic: A longitudinal probability sample survey of the UK population. *Lancet Psychiatry* **2020**, *7*, 883–892. [CrossRef]
17. Wong, L.P.; Alias, H.; Md Fuzi, A.A.; Omar, I.S.; Mohamad Nor, A.; Tan, M.P.; Baranovich, D.L.; Saari, C.Z.; Hamzah, S.H.; Cheong, K.W.; et al. Escalating progression of mental health disorders during the COVID-19 pandemic: Evidence from a nationwide survey. *PLoS ONE* **2021**, *16*, e0248916. [CrossRef] [PubMed]
18. Priola, V.; Pecis, L. Missing voices: The absence of women from Italy's COVID-19 pandemic response. *Gend. Manag.* **2020**, *35*, 619–627. [CrossRef]
19. Wenham, C.; Smith, J.; Davies, S.E.; Feng, H.; Grépin, K.A.; Harman, S.; Herten-Crabb, A.; Morgan, R. Women are most affected by pandemics—Lessons from past outbreaks. *Nature* **2020**, *583*, 194–198. [CrossRef]
20. Jin, J.-M.; Bai, P.; He, W.; Wu, F.; Liu, X.-F.; Han, D.-M.; Liu, S.; Yang, J.-K. Gender differences in patients with COVID-19: Focus on severity and mortality. *Front. Public Health* **2020**, *8*, 152. [CrossRef]
21. Del Boca, D.; Oggero, N.; Profeta, P.; Rossi, M. Women's and men's work, housework and childcare, before and during COVID-19. *Rev. Econ. Househ.* **2020**, *18*, 1001–1017. [CrossRef] [PubMed]
22. Proto, E.; Quintana-Domeque, C. COVID-19 and mental health deterioration by ethnicity and gender in the UK. *PLoS ONE* **2021**, *16*, e0244419. [CrossRef] [PubMed]
23. Xue, B.; McMunn, A. Gender differences in unpaid care work and psychological distress in the UK COVID-19 lockdown. *PLoS ONE* **2021**, *16*, e0247959. [CrossRef] [PubMed]
24. Del Río-Casanova, L.; Sánchez-Martín, M.; García-Dantas, A.; González-Vázquez, A.; Justo, A. Psychological Responses According to Gender during the Early Stage of COVID-19 in Spain. *Int. J. Environ. Res. Public Health* **2021**, *18*, 3731. [CrossRef]

25. Yan, S.; Xu, R.; Stratton, T.D.; Kavcic, V.; Luo, D.; Hou, F.; Bi, F.; Jiao, R.; Song, K.; Jiang, Y. Sex differences and psychological stress: Responses to the COVID-19 pandemic in China. *BMC Public Health* **2021**, *21*, 79. [CrossRef]
26. Yoshioka, T.; Okubo, R.; Tabuchi, T.; Odani, S.; Shinozaki, T.; Tsugawa, Y. Factors associated with serious psychological distress during the COVID-19 pandemic in Japan: A nationwide cross-sectional internet-based study. *BMJ Open* **2021**, *11*, e051115. [CrossRef]
27. Di Blasi, M.; Gullo, S.; Mancinelli, E.; Freda, M.F.; Esposito, G.; Gelo, O.C.G.; Lagetto, G.; Giordano, C.; Mazzeschi, C.; Pazzagli, C.; et al. Psychological distress associated with the COVID-19 lockdown: A two-wave network analysis. *J. Affect. Disord.* **2021**, *284*, 18–26. [CrossRef]
28. Tyra, A.T.; Griffin, S.M.; Fergus, T.A.; Ginty, A.T. Individual differences in emotion regulation prospectively predict early COVID-19 related acute stress. *J. Anxiety Disord.* **2021**, *81*, 102411. [CrossRef]
29. Parra-Rizo, M.A.; Sanchís-Soler, G. Physical Activity and the Improvement of Autonomy, Functional Ability, Subjective Health, and Social Relationships in Women over the Age of 60. *Int. J. Environ. Res. Public Health* **2021**, *18*, 6926. [CrossRef]
30. Anderson, E.C.; Carleton, R.N.; Diefenbach, M.; Han, P.K. The relationship between uncertainty and affect. *Front. Psychol.* **2019**, *10*, 2504. [CrossRef]
31. Carleton, R.N. Into the unknown: A review and synthesis of contemporary models involving uncertainty. *J. Anxiety Disord.* **2016**, *39*, 30–43. [CrossRef]
32. Shu, J.; Ochsner, K.; Phelps, E.A. The Impact of Intolerance of Uncertainty on Reappraisal and Suppression. Available online: https://psyarxiv.com/fsnvy (accessed on 27 September 2021). [CrossRef]
33. Prati, G. Mental health and its psychosocial predictors during national quarantine in Italy against the coronavirus disease 2019 (COVID-19). *Anxiety Stress Coping* **2021**, *34*, 145–156. [CrossRef]
34. Lovibond, P.F.; Lovibond, S.H. The structure of negative emotional states: Comparison of the depression anxiety stress scales (DASS) with the Beck Depression and Anxiety Inventories. *Behav. Res. Ther.* **1995**, *33*, 335–343. [CrossRef]
35. Bottesi, G.; Ghisi, M.; Altoè, G.; Conforti, E.; Melli, G.; Soca, C. The Italian version of the Depression, Anxiety and Stress Scale-21: Factor structure and psychometric properties on community and clinical samples. *Compr. Psychiatry* **2015**, *60*, 170–181. [CrossRef]
36. Gross, J.J.; John, O.P. Individual differences in two emotion regulation processes: Implications for affect, relationships, and well-being. *J. Pers. Soc. Psychol.* **2003**, *85*, 348–362. [CrossRef] [PubMed]
37. Balzarotti, S.; John, O.P.; Gross, J.J. An Italian adaptation of the emotion regulation questionnaire. *Eur. J. Psychol. Assess.* **2010**, *26*, 61–67. [CrossRef]
38. Carleton, R.N.; Norton, P.J. Asmundson GJG. Fearing the unknown: A short version of the Intolerance of Uncertainty Scale. *J. Anxiety Disord.* **2007**, *21*, 105–117. [CrossRef] [PubMed]
39. Lauriola, M.; Mosca, O.; Carleton, R.N. Hierarchical factor structure of the intolerance of uncertainty scale short form (ius-12) in the Italian version. *TPM Testing* **2016**, *23*, 377–394. [CrossRef]
40. Clark, L.A.; Watson, D. Constructing validity: Basic issues in objective scale development. *Psychol. Assess.* **1995**, *7*, 309–319. [CrossRef]
41. Nunnally, J. *Psychometric Theory*, 2nd ed.; McGraw-Hill: New York, NY, USA, 1978.
42. Hair, J.F.; Black, W.C.; Babin, B.J.; Anderson, R.E.; Tatham, R.L. *Multivariate Data Analysis*, 6th ed.; Pearson University Press: Upper Saddle River, NJ, USA, 2006.
43. Lorant, V.; Smith, P.; Van den Broeck, K.; Nicaise, P. Psychological distress associated with the COVID-19 pandemic and suppression measures during the first wave in Belgium. *BMC Psychiatry* **2021**, *21*, 1–10. [CrossRef]
44. Shevlin, M.; McBride, O.; Murphy, J.; Miller, J.G.; Hartman, T.K.; Levita, L.; Mason, L.; Martinez, A.P.; McKay, R.; Stocks, T.; et al. Anxiety, depression, traumatic stress and COVID-19-related anxiety in the UK general population during the COVID-19 pandemic. *BJPsych Open* **2020**, *6*, e125. [CrossRef] [PubMed]
45. Frank, P.; Lob, E.; Steptoe, A.; Fancourt, D. Trajectories of depressive symptoms among vulnerable groups in the UK during the COVID-19 pandemic. *medRxiv* 2020. [CrossRef]
46. Fisher, A.N.; Ryan, M.K. Gender inequalities during COVID-19. *Group Process. Intergroup. Relat.* **2021**, *24*, 237–245. [CrossRef]
47. Brans, K.; Koval, P.; Verduyn, P.; Lim, Y.L.; Kuppens, P. The regulation of negative and positive affect in daily life. *Emotion* **2013**, *13*, 926–939. [CrossRef]
48. Richardson, C.M.E. Emotion regulation in the context of daily stress: Impact on daily affect. *Pers. Individ. Differ.* **2017**, *112*, 150–156. [CrossRef]
49. Hu, T.; Zhang, D.; Wang, J.; Mistry, R.; Ran, G.; Wang, X. Relation between emotion regulation and mental health: A meta-analysis review. *Psychol. Rep.* **2014**, *114*, 341–362. [CrossRef] [PubMed]
50. Khantzian, E.J. The self-medication hypothesis of substance use disorders: A reconsideration and recent applications. *Harv. Rev. Psychiatry* **1997**, *4*, 231–244. [CrossRef] [PubMed]
51. Wang, K.; Goldenberg, A.; Dorison, C.A.; Miller, J.K.; Uusberg, A.; Lerner, J.S.; Isager, P.M. A multi-country test of brief reappraisal interventions on emotions during the COVID-19 pandemic. *Nat. Hum. Behav.* **2021**, *5*, 1089–1110. [CrossRef]

52. Moducci, R. "Attività conoscitiva preliminare all'esame del documento di economia e finanza 2020", Presented at V Commissione "Bilancio, tesoro e programmazione" della Camera dei Deputati 5a Commissione "Bilancio" del Senato della Repubblica Roma, 28 April. Available online: www.istat.it/it/files//2020/04/Istat_Audizione-DEF_28aprile2020.pdf (accessed on 31 October 2021).
53. Mazza, C.; Marchetti, D.; Ricci, E.; Fontanesi, L.; Di Giandomenico, S.; Verrocchio, M.C.; Roma, P. The COVID-19 lockdown and psychological distress among Italian parents: Influence of parental role, parent personality, and child difficulties. *Int. J. Psychol.* **2021**, *56*, 577–584. [CrossRef] [PubMed]
54. Etheridge, B.; Spantig, L. *The Gender Gap in Mental Well-Being during the COVID-19 Outbreak: Evidence from the UK (No. 2020-08)*; ISER Working Paper Series; ISER: Essex, UK, 2020.

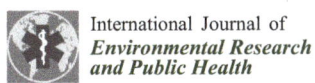

Article

Health-Related Quality of Life of Elderly Women with Fall Experiences

Jiyoung Song [1] and Eunwon Lee [2],*

1 College of Nursing, Korea University, Seoul 02841, Korea; nav857@naver.com
2 Department of Nursing, Gwangju University, Jinwol-dong, Gwangju-si 61743, Korea
* Correspondence: ewlee@gwangju.ac.kr; Tel.: +82-62-670-2377

Abstract: This study aimed to describe the health-related quality of life of elderly women with experience in fall treatment as well as to prepare basic data for the development of interventions to improve the quality of life for this group. The study was based on raw data from the 2019 Korea Community Health Survey. Using the SPSS program, the characteristics of the subjects were tested by frequency, percentage, and chi-square test. To establish the impact of fall experience on the health-related quality of life of elderly women, the OR and 95% CI were calculated using multiple logistic regression analysis. Of the 4260 people surveyed, 44.7% of the elderly women said they had a high quality of life, whereas 55.3% of the elderly women said they had a low quality of life. A younger age was associated with a better-rated health-related quality of life. Those who lived in a city and had a high level of education tended to describe a high quality of life. The quality of life was considered high by those who exercised, but low by those who were obese or diabetic. The results of this study can lead to a better understanding of the experiences of elderly women who have experienced falls, and they can be used as basic data for the development of related health programs.

Keywords: fall; women; health-related quality of life; South Korea

1. Introduction

Falls are commonly occurring accidents in older people, and they have become an important health issue as the number of older people increases with the aging population [1,2]. Over the past year, 15.9% of Korea's elderly experienced falls, with the fall rate of female seniors recorded at 19.4%, higher than that of male seniors at 11.2%; the hospital utilization rate was also reported to be high [3].

Falls have a wide range of effects from minor accidents to serious injuries and deaths [4], and they also affect the person's emotional state, degrading the overall quality of life via a loss of confidence and increased social isolation [5,6]. In practice, falls are a predictable and preventable problem in more than 70% of cases; thus, the expansion of social awareness [7] toward the identification of fall risk factors should enable fall prevention arbitration [8]. According to the growth trend of the elderly population, the threat to health and quality of life caused by falls and the socioeconomic costs are expected to further increase in the future; thus, falls could also become a socioeconomic problem [9,10]. Addressing falls in older adults requires a broad understanding of the integrated assessment of various aspects such as balance, depression, and quality of life [11]. Falls are complicated and considered important factors that reduce the quality of life of older adults [5,6].

Health-related Quality of life (HRQoL) can be defined as the subjective satisfaction with life in the physical, psychological, spiritual, and socioeconomic areas [12,13], which becomes more of an issue as life expectancy increases [14]. Factors affecting the health-related quality of life of the elderly include gender, socioeconomic level, physical and mental health, performance of daily life activities, subjective health status, and health behaviors [15–17]. In particular, many studies [1,11,18] have found that women's health-related quality of life is lower than that of men. After the death of the spouse, the elderly woman has a more difficult time than men due to problems such as health, poverty, and depression [18].

Various factors affect the health-related quality of life (HRQoL) of elderly women [11]. It decreases with increasing age, low income, or living alone and low education [17,18]. Additionally, it is low in individuals with chronic diseases, such as high blood pressure and diabetes, depression, and those taking long-term medication [19,20]. Furthermore, HRQoL is low in patients with decreased muscle mass, high BMI, and limited physical activity [15,17], and health behaviors, such as drinking, smoking, and exercise, affect HRQoL [1,18]. Park [12] found that the four variables of depression, physical function, health level, and regular exercise encompass 26% of the variance in women's HRQoL.

Studies related to health-related quality of life have been conducted in older adults [15,16] and in patients with certain diseases such as diabetes [19,20]. In the current situation in which the elderly population is increasing, it is necessary to learn about the health-related quality of life of elderly women, who are known to experience more falls and have a lower quality of life than men. In this study, we used raw data from the Korea Community Health Survey [21] to examine the health-related quality of life of female senior citizens with experience in fall treatment as well as to prepare basic data for the development of interventions to improve the quality of life.

2. Materials and Methods

2.1. Study Design and Study Participants

This study was a descriptive research study that used the 2019 Korea Community Health Survey (KCHS) [21] to identify the health-related quality of life according to the fall experiences of elderly women. The KCHS was conducted at 255 health centers nationwide, beginning in 2008, for adults aged 19 or older, to produce comparable regional health statistics to formulate and evaluate regional healthcare plans. In order to collect data, trained investigators visited selected sample households, provided explanations for the investigation and confidentiality to the person surveyed, and received consent to participate. One-to-one interviews were conducted using electronic survey computer-assisted personal interviewing.

Of the 229,099 participants who participated in the 2019 Community Health Survey, elderly women aged ≥65 years with experience of falling treatment were included in this study. The exclusion criteria were men, aged <65 years, no falling treatment experiences, and missing related questionnaire replies (HRQoL, health behaviors, and health-related questions). In this study, fall experience was defined as the presence of fall over the past one year. 'Have you fallen in the last year (including slips, flips)?' The single question identified the experience of fall. Finally, a total of 4260 participants were included in the analysis (Figure 1).

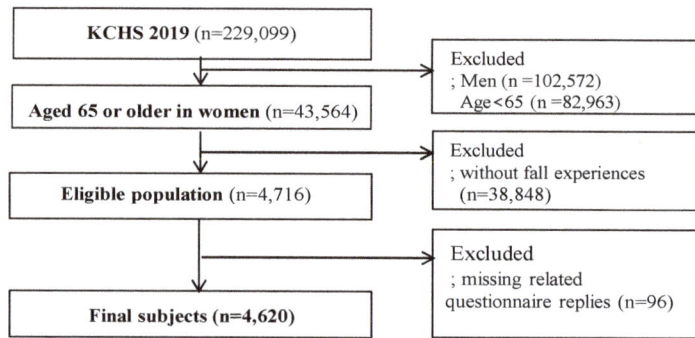

Figure 1. The criteria for inclusion and exclusion of participants.

2.2. Study Variables

2.2.1. Demographic Characteristics

The demographic characteristics of the subjects used data on age (65–69, 70–79, ≥80), area of residence, level of education, and marriage status. The general characteristics were modified to suit the purpose of this study, based on the literature review [8,10,18]. The area of residence was divided into towns and villages. The level of education was categorized as "no studies", "elementary-school graduation", "middle-school graduation", and "high-school graduation". The marriage status was divided into no spouse (including divorce, bereavement, separation, and unmarried) and having a spouse.

2.2.2. HRQoL

Health-related quality of life was established by the Euro-Qol Group [22] and measured using the Korean version of EQ-5D-3L (EuroQoL-5D), which is widely used to measure quality of life [23]. The EQ-5D index consists of five subindexes: mobility (M), self-care (SC), daily activities (UA), pain and discomfort (PD), and anxiety and depression (AD). In this study, the weighting of the Korea Centers for Disease Control and Prevention (KCDC), which expresses health status as a value from –0.171 to 1 in consideration of the characteristics of Koreans, was applied. The weights were as follows:

$$EQ\_5D = 1 - (0.05 + 0.096 \times M2 + 0.418 \times M3 + 0.046 \times SC2 + 0.136 \times SC3 + 0.051 \times UA2 + 0.208 \times UA3 \\ + 0.037 \times PD2 + 0.151 \times PD3 + 0.043 \times AD2 + 0.158A \times D3 + 0.05 \times N3). \quad (1)$$

In particular, this study distinguished between high and low quality of life using an EQ-5D index threshold of 60% to determine the health-related quality of life of elderly women with experience in fall treatment.

2.2.3. Health Behavior Characteristics

Health behavior characteristics included smoking, drinking, exercising, and sleeping. Based on the literature review [8,10,18], the health behavior characteristics were modified to suit the purpose of this study. Smoking behavior was categorized into current nonsmokers who had never smoked ordinary cigarettes in their lives, a smoking cessation group who had smoked in the past but did not smoke at the point of data collection, a smoking group who smoked every day, and a smoking group who smoked sometimes. Drinking behavior was categorized into a nondrinking group if alcohol had not been consumed in the past year, or a drinking group if it had been consumed. Exercise was positively defined if it occurred more than once in the past week (days when the body had more than 10 min of intense physical activity leading to more difficult breathing than usual). Sleep was categorized on the basis of the number of hours of sleep per day, divided into groups of 0 to 7 h and more than 8 h.

2.2.4. Physical Health

Physical health characteristics included obesity, hypertension, and diabetes. Obesity was defined as BMI (kg/m^2) >30; otherwise, BMI was considered normal [18]. Hypertension and diabetes were based on a doctor's diagnosis [21].

2.3. Data Analysis

Data analysis was carried out using the IBM SPSS statistics 23.0 program. Since the community health survey samples were collected under a complex sampling design, a composite sample plan file reflecting stratified variables, colonies, and weights was generated according to the data analysis guidelines of the Korea Disease Control and Prevention Agency, and then, a composite sample analysis was undertaken. The characteristics of demographic factors, health behaviors, and physical health were described using frequency and percentage. Overall differences in proportions between groups were analyzed with the chi-square test. The HRQoL scores according to each variable were presented as the mean ± standard error using *t*-test and ANOVAs. In order to determine the effects of demographics, health behavior, and physical health on the health-related quality of life in older women with experience in fall treatment, multiple logistic regression analysis was conducted. Each odds ratio (OR) was reported together with its 95% confidence interval (CI). All statistical significance levels were set at $p < 0.05$.

2.4. Ethical Considerations

The Community Health Survey is a government-designated statistical tool based on Article 17 of the Statistics Act (Approved No. 117015). The Korea Centers for Disease Control and Prevention provide only unidentified data so that individuals cannot be identified from the survey data. The raw data used in this study were requested from the Korea Disease Control and Prevention Agency (https://chs.kdca.go.kr/chs/index.do, accessed on 25 March 2021) and received through the approval process for use. The research was conducted after receiving an exemption from the Public Institutional Review Board of the Ministry of Health and Welfare (IRB No.: P01-202103-22-008).

3. Results

3.1. Characteristics of Elderly Women According to Health-Related Quality of Life

Group demographic characteristics, physical health, and health behavioral factors are shown in Table 1; 55.3% of the elderly women included in this study ($n = 4260$) considered their quality of life (QoL) to be low. There was a significant difference in age, residence, education, spouse presence, smoking, drinking, exercise, obesity, hypertension, and diabetes between low and high QoL groups ($p < 0.001$); 27.2% of the individuals who reported drinking said their QoL was low, while 24.9% said their QoL was high ($p = 0.049$). In terms of sleep duration, 82.8% and 17.2% of the elderly who slept 0–7 h and >8 h per night, respectively, said they had a high QoL; however, this difference did not reach significance ($p = 0.053$).

Table 1. Characteristics of elderly women according to HRQoL ($n = 4260$).

Variables	Categories	Low (n = 2355) n (%)	High (n = 1905) n (%)	p
Age	65–69	307 (13.9)	594 (33.1)	<0.001
	70–79	1151 (50.9)	968 (50.8)	
	≥80	897 (35.2)	343 (16.1)	
Residence	City	878 (68.7)	858 (76.7)	<0.001
	Town	1477 (31.3)	1047 (23.3)	
Education	No	873 (29.3)	416 (14.2)	<0.001
	Elementary school	1105 (45.2)	894 (41.4)	
	Middle school	216 (12.8)	320 (21.9)	
	≥High school	161 (12.7)	275 (22.5)	
With husband	No	1514 (61.6)	973 (50.1)	<0.001
	Yes	841 (38.4)	932 (49.9)	
Smoking	Nonsmoker	2222 (93.9)	1834 (96.0)	<0.001
	Quit	85 (3.4)	37 (2.0)	
	Yes	48 (2.6)	34 (2.0)	
Drinking	No	1740 (72.8)	1465 (75.1)	0.049
	Yes	615 (27.2)	440 (24.9)	
Exercise	No	2199 (94.9)	1667 (87.3)	<0.001
	Yes	156 (5.1)	238 (12.7)	

Table 1. Cont.

Variables	Categories	Low (n = 2355) n (%)	High (n = 1905) n (%)	p
Sleep duration (h)	0–7	1854 (81.0)	1521 (82.8)	0.053
	≥8	501 (19.0)	384 (17.2)	
Obese	No	2177 (93.0)	1819 (95.8)	<0.001
	Yes	178 (7.0)	86 (4.2)	
Hypertension	No	824 (35.4)	847 (43.7)	<0.001
	Yes	1531 (64.6)	1058 (56.3)	
DM	No	1732 (70.9)	1498 (77.0)	<0.001
	Yes	623 (29.1)	407 (23.0)	

3.2. HRQoL According to Characteristics of Elderly Women

HRQoL, according to demographic, health behavior, and physical health characteristics of elderly women, is shown in Table 2. The HRQoL score was significantly different as a function of age, living area, education level, spouse presence, smoking, drinking, exercise, sleep, obesity, hypertension, and diabetes ($p < 0.001$). Women who were younger, lived in cities, had a higher level of education, and had a spouse had higher HRQoL scores ($p < 0.001$). Additionally, HRQoL was higher in individuals who did not smoke or drink and regularly exercised. Older women with obesity, diabetes, and hypertension had lower HRQoL scores ($p < 0.001$). In terms of sleep duration, the QoL of elderly women who slept 0–7 h per night was 0.77 ± 0.00, which was higher than in those women who slept >8 h (0.76 ± 0.01; $p = 0.014$).

Table 2. HRQoL according to characteristics of elderly women (n = 4260).

Variables	Categories	Mean ± SE	p
Age	65–69	0.85 ± 0.00	<0.001
	70–79	0.78 ± 0.00	
	≥80	0.71 ± 0.00	
Residence	City	0.79 ± 0.00	<0.001
	Town	0.76 ± 0.00	
Education	No	0.72 ± 0.01	<0.001
	Elementary school	0.77 ± 0.00	
	Middle school	0.82 ± 0.01	
	≥High school	0.83 ± 0.01	
With husband	No	0.76 ± 0.00	<0.001
	Yes	0.80 ± 0.00	
Smoking	Nonsmoker	0.77 ± 0.00	<0.001
	Quit	0.70 ± 0.01	
	Yes	0.75 ± 0.02	
Drinking	No	0.77 ± 0.00	<0.001
	Yes	0.75 ± 0.01	
Sleep duration (h)	0–7	0.77 ± 0.00	0.014
	≥8	0.76 ± 0.01	
Exercise	No	0.76 ± 0.00	<0.001
	Yes	0.83 ± 0.00	
Obese	No	0.78 ± 0.00	<0.001
	Yes	0.73 ± 0.01	
Hypertension	No	0.80 ± 0.00	<0.001
	Yes	0.76 ± 0.00	
DM	No	0.78 ± 0.00	<0.001
	Yes	0.74 ± 0.01	

Mean ± SE: mean ± standard error.

3.3. Factors Affecting Health-Related QoL in Elderly Women

The results of examining the effects of demographic, health behavior, and physical health characteristics of elderly women on health-related quality of life are shown in Table 3.

Table 3. Factors affecting HRQoL in elderly women (*n* = 4260).

Variables	Categories	OR	95% CI
Age	65–69	1	
	70–79	0.51 ***	0.45–0.58
	≥80	0.27 ***	0.23–0.32
Residence	City	1	
	Town	0.81 ***	0.74–0.89
Education	No	1	
	Elementary school	1.43 ***	1.24–1.66
	Middle school	2.19 ***	1.81–2.65
	≥High school	2.20 ***	1.81–2.68
With husband	No	1	
	Yes	1.04	0.93–1.17
Smoking	Nonsmoker	1	
	Quit	0.58 ***	0.42–0.80
	Yes	0.72 ***	0.52–0.98
Drinking	No	1	
	Yes	0.94	0.82–1.07
Exercise	No	1	
	Yes	2.18 ***	1.87–2.54
Sleep duration	0–7	1	
	≥8	1.06	0.93–1.20
Obese	No	1	
	Yes	0.60 ***	0.48–0.75
Hypertension	No	1	
	Yes	0.90	0.80–1.01
DM	No	1	
	Yes	0.79 ***	0.69–0.91

OR: odds ratio; CI: confidence interval; *** $p < 0.001$.

Compared with women aged 65 to 69, women aged 70 to 79 had 0.51-fold (95% CI: 0.45–0.58) and women aged 80 or older had 0.27-fold (95% CI: 0.23–0.32) lower HRQoL scores. Compared with elderly women living in urban areas, the health-related QoL score of elderly women living in rural areas was 0.81-fold higher (95% CI: 0.74–0.89). At the educational level, the health-related quality of life score for elementary-school graduates was 1.43-fold higher (95% CI: 1.24–1.66), for middle-school graduates was 2.19-fold higher (95% CI: 1.81–2.65), and for high-school graduates was 2.20-fold higher (95% CI: 1.81–2.68) than that of elderly women with no education. In terms of marital status, the health-related quality of life score for elderly women with spouses was 1.04-fold (95% CI: 0.93–1.17) higher than that of elderly women without spouses.

In the case of smoking, the health-related quality of life score of elderly women in the smoking cessation group was 0.58-fold lower (95% CI: 0.42–0.80) and the HRQoL of smokers was 0.72-fold lower (95% CI: 0.52–0.98) than that of nonsmokers. In the case of drinking, the health-related quality of life of the drinking group was 0.94-fold (95% CI: 0.82–1.07) lower compared with the nondrinking group. Elderly women who exercised had a 2.18-fold higher (95% CI: 1.87–2.54) HRQoL score compared with elderly women who did not exercise. With respect to sleep duration, the health-related QoL score of elderly women who sleep more than 8 h was 1.06-fold higher (95% CI: 0.93 to 1.20) than that of elderly women who slept 0 to 7 h.

Compared with nonobese elderly women in this study, the health-related quality of life score of obese elderly women was 0.60-fold lower (95% CI: 0.48–0.75). The health-related quality of life score in elderly women diagnosed with hypertension was 0.90-fold lower (95% CI: 0.81–1.01) than that of undiagnosed elderly women, whereas this proportion was 0.79-fold lower (95% CI: 0.69–0.91) in elderly women diagnosed with diabetes compared with undiagnosed elderly women.

4. Discussion

Using raw data from the Korea Community Health Survey, this study sought to determine the quality of life related to health of elderly women with experience in fall treatment. Of the 4260 people surveyed, 44.7% said they had a high quality of life while 55.3% said they had a low quality of life. According to the results of several previous studies [5,6], health-related quality of life is found to be lower in those who experienced falls; however, in this study, health-related quality of life was only evaluated for elderly women with fall treatment experience. In addition, quality of life was distinguished as high or low according to an EQ-5D index threshold of 60%, which will require repeated research in the future.

In the comparison of elderly women with a high quality of life and those with a low quality of life, there were significant differences in all variables except for sleep time. In accordance with the findings of [17,18], quality of life decreased with age. The increase in the number of falls and the degree of injuries with increasing age was not considered, but we were able to identify age as an influential factor on quality of life. Quality of life is accepted as subjective wellbeing and satisfaction with life; the elderly typically exhibit the lowest life satisfaction, warranting increased attention. According to this study, elderly women living in cities had a higher quality of life than elderly women living in rural areas, who exhibited scores that were 0.81-fold lower (95% CI: 0.74–0.89). Studies in other countries have also reported high health-related life scores in socioeconomically developed regions [24]. In this sense, facilities frequently used by senior citizens, such as medical institutions and welfare centers, need to be prepared without regional bias.

In agreement with previous studies [16,24], a higher educational background led to a higher quality of life. It is thought that people with high educational standards perceive a higher quality of life due to their socioeconomic affluence and health activities. As such, continuous education related to hobbies is recommended for senior citizens at welfare centers. In this study, marriage status did not affect the quality of life of elderly women; in another study [25], it was found that marriage status affected the health-related lives of men but not women. Further research is required in this regard.

A previous study of middle-aged women found that smoking had a high influence on the health-related quality of life [26], whereas another study found that smoking did not affect quality of life in older people [18]. In this study, the health-related quality of life of elderly women in the smoking cessation group was 0.58-fold lower (95% CI: 0.42–0.80) and that of elderly smokers was 0.72-fold lower (95% CI: 0.52–0.98) than that of nonsmokers. The number of elderly smokers in this study was small; thus, the generalizability of these results is limited. Additional studies will be needed in the future, in which the entire population can be divided into smoking, smoking cessation, and nonsmoking groups. In terms of drinking alcohol, a previous study mentioned that only drinking volume affects quality of life [27], but this study did not elucidate the factors affecting quality of life. Further studies will be needed to distinguish the amount, frequency, and type of alcohol to establish the impact of drinking on quality of life. In this study, the quality of life of elderly women who exercised was 2.18-fold (95% CI: 1.87–2.54) higher than that of those who did not exercise, in line with previous studies [28,29]. Exercise has the effect of increasing muscle strength to prevent falls, as well as improving quality of life; therefore, it should be actively recommended for elderly women. In addition, it is agreed that frequent walking leads to a higher quality of life, despite it not being a complex form of exercise; thus, various walking programs should be established in the community [1].

In agreement with [1,18], the health-related quality of life of obese women was found to be low in this study. To prevent obesity, in addition to proper exercise, regulated dietary intake and proper eating habits are necessary. It was previously reported that quality of life decreases upon diagnosis of a chronic disease [6,25]. In this study, the quality of life of elderly women diagnosed with diabetes was 0.79-fold lower (95% CI: 0.69–0.91) than that of elderly women not diagnosed. The HRQoL of elderly people with diabetes is directly affected by the dysfunction caused by aging [20], which requires appropriate nursing intervention. It has been reported that a higher number of accompanying diseases leads to a lower quality of life [25]; therefore, in the future, various studies will need to be conducted to consider the type, number, treatment period, and complications of chronic diseases [18].

In this study, we found various factors that affected the HRQoL of elderly women; however, it is important to prevent falls before they occur. Considering these points, it is necessary to improve the socio-physical environment of the elderly and predict the risk of falling by assessing their sense of balance in advance [30]. In addition, research and educational programs should be developed by creating a database of fall risk factors [31].

The investigation of factors affecting the QoL of elderly women with experiences of fall treatment using community health surveys can provide a source of basic data for the development of health-related programs in the future. However, this study has some limitations. It has a cross-sectional design using secondary data, and it is difficult to explain the temporal context of the older women with fall experiences and their related factors. In addition, this study was conducted without considering other diseases, the time of the fall, treatment period, injury area, and surgery of older women in detail. Therefore, further studies are required that would consider the physical, mental health, and environment factors affecting older women.

5. Conclusions

This study investigated the factors affecting the health-related quality of life of elderly women with experience of fall treatment using the Korea Community Health Survey. Among 4260 participants, 44.7% considered their quality of life to be high and 55.3% considered their quality of life to be low. Younger respondents had a better health-related quality of life. Those who lived in a city and had a high level of education also considered their quality of life to be high. A high HRQoL was reported by elderly women who exercised, whereas a low HRQoL was reported by obese or diabetic women. This study is fragmentary in that it is not possible to grasp the context of the effect of fall treatment experience on HRQoL. However, it is significant in that it used a community health survey as a representative sample of Korea. The results of this study allow a better understanding of the elderly who have experienced falls and can be used as a source of basic data for the development of related health programs.

Author Contributions: Conceptualization, J.S.; methodology, J.S.; validation, E.L.; formal analysis, J.S.; writing—original draft preparation, J.S.; writing—review and editing, E.L. All authors have read and agreed to the published version of the manuscript.

Funding: This research received no external funding.

Institutional Review Board Statement: The study was conducted according to the guidelines of the Declaration of Helsinki, and approved an exemption by the Institutional Review Board of the Ministry of Health and Welfare (IRB No.: P01-202103-22-008).

Informed Consent Statement: Informed consent was obtained from all subjects involved in the study.

Data Availability Statement: The data presented in this study are available upon request from the Korea Disease Control and Prevention Agency (KDCA). The request for data can be found here: https://chs.kdca.go.kr/chs/index.do (accessed on 25 March 2021).

Conflicts of Interest: The authors declare no conflict of interest.

References

1. Gouveia, B.R.; Ihle, A.; Kliegel, M.; Freitas, D.L.; Gouveia, É.R. Sex differences in relation patterns between health-related quality of life of older adults and its correlates: A population-based cross-sectional study in Madeira, Portugal. *Prim. Health Care Res. Dev.* **2018**, *20*, 1–5. [CrossRef]
2. Kang, Y.O.; Song, R.Y. Validation of Fall Risk Assessment Scales among Hospitalized Patients in South Korea Using Retrospective Data Analysis. *Korean J. Adult Nurs.* **2015**, *27*, 29–38. [CrossRef]
3. Ministry of Health and Welfare (MOHW). *2017 Korean National Survey on Older Adults*; MOHW: Sejong, Korean, 2017. Available online: http://www.mohw.go.kr/react/jb/sjb030301vw.jsp (accessed on 25 March 2021).
4. World Health Organization (WHO). *WHO Global Report on Falls Prevention in Older Age*; WHO: Geneva, Switzerland, 2007. Available online: https://www.who.int/ageing/publications/Falls_prevention7March.pdf?ua=1 (accessed on 25 March 2021).
5. Jeon, M.J.; Jeon, H.S.; Yi, C.H.; Cynn, H.S. Comparison of Elderly Fallers and Elderly Non-Fallers: Balancing Ability, Depression, and Quality of Life. *Phys. Ther. Korea* **2014**, *21*, 45–54. [CrossRef]
6. Thiem, U.; Klaaßen-Mielke, R.; Trampisch, U.; Moschny, A.; Pientka, L.; Hinrichs, T. Falls and EQ-5D rated quality of life in community-dwelling seniors with concurrent chronic diseases: A cross-sectional study. *Health Qual. Life Outcomes* **2014**, *12*, 1–7. [CrossRef]
7. Park, H.O.; Kang, H.K. A Literature Review for Fall-Prevention Nursing Program Development based on the Fall Information of a Rehabilitation Hospital. *J. Converg. Inf. Technol.* **2020**, *10*, 99–107. [CrossRef]
8. White, A.M.; Tooth, L.R.; Peeters, G.G. Fall Risk Factors in Mid-Age Women: The Australian Longitudinal Study on Women's Health. *Am. J. Prev. Med.* **2018**, *54*, 51–63. [CrossRef]
9. Park, N.J.; Shin, Y.S. Predictors of Accidental Falls in the Community-dwelling Elderly by Age. *J. Korean Acad. Community Health Nurs.* **2019**, *30*, 141–149. [CrossRef]
10. Sibley, K.M.; Voth, J.; Munce, S.E.; Straus, S.E.; Jaglal, S.B. Chronic disease and falls in community-dwelling Canadians over 65 years old: A population-based study exploring associations with number and pattern of chronic conditions. *BMC Geriatr.* **2014**, *14*, 22. [CrossRef]
11. Maranesi, E.; Fioretti, S.; Ghetti, G.G.; Rabini, R.A.; Burattini, L.; Mercante, O.; Di Nardo, F. The surface electromyographic evaluation of the Functional Reach in elderly subjects. *J. Electromyogr. Kinesiol.* **2016**, *26*, 102–110. [CrossRef]
12. Park, J.M.; Kim, C.S.; Kim, M.W. A Path Analysis on Factors—Depression, Level of Health status, Physical Function, and Regular Exercise—Influencing Health Related Quality of Life according to sex in Community dwelling Elderly. *J. Korean Public Health Nurs.* **2016**, *30*, 337–348. [CrossRef]
13. Pilar, P.R.; Francisco, M.M. EQ-5D-3L for Assessing Quality of Life in Older Nursing Home Residents with Cognitive Impairment. *Life* **2020**, *10*, 100. [CrossRef]
14. Jang, S.H.; Yeum, D.M. Analysis of the Types and Affecting Factors of Older People's Health-related Quality of Life, Using Latent Class Analysis. *J. Korean Acad. Community Health Nurs.* **2020**, *31*, 212–221. [CrossRef]
15. Leirós-Rodríguez, R.; Romo-Pérez, V.; García-Soidán, J.L.; Soto-Rodríguez, A. Prevalence and Factors Associated with Functional Limitations during Aging in a Representative Sample of Spanish Population. *Phys. Occup. Ther. Geriatr.* **2018**, *36*, 156–167. [CrossRef]
16. Moon, S.M. Gender differences in the impact of socioeconomic, health-related, and health behavioral factors on the health-related quality of life of the Korean elderly. *J. Digit. Converg.* **2017**, *15*, 259–271. [CrossRef]
17. Janssen, M.F.; Szende, A.; Cabases, J.; Ramos-Goñi, J.M.; Vilagut, G. Population norms for the EQ-5D-3L: A cross-country analysis of population surveys for 20 countries. *Eur. J. Health Econ.* **2019**, *20*, 205–216. [CrossRef] [PubMed]
18. Oh, H.S. Important significant factors of health-related quality of life (EQ-5D) by age group in Korea based on KNHANES (2014). *J. Korean Data Inf. Sci. Soc.* **2017**, *28*, 573–584. [CrossRef]
19. Alefishat, E.S.; Jarab, A.; Abu, F.R. Factors affecting health-related quality of life among hypertensive patients using the EQ-5D tool. *Int. J. Clin. Pract.* **2020**, *74*, e13532. [CrossRef]
20. Maranesi, E.; Di Nardo, F.; Rabini, R.A.A.; Ghetti, G.G.G.; Burattini, L.; Mercante, O. Muscle activation patterns related to diabetic neuropathy in elderly subjects: A Functional Reach Test study. *Clin. Biomech.* **2015**, *32*, 236–240. [CrossRef]
21. Korea Disease Control and Prevention Agency. *2019 Community Health Survey*; Korea Disease Control and Prevention Agency: Cheongju, Korea, 2019. Available online: https://chs.cdc.go.kr/chs/rawDta/rawDtaProvdMain.do (accessed on 1 August 2020).
22. The EuroQol Group. EuroQol—A new facility for the measurement of health-related quality of life. *Health Policy* **1990**, *16*, 199–208. [CrossRef]
23. Lee, Y.; Nam, H.; Chuang, L.; Kim, K.; Yang, H.; Kwon, I. South Korean Time Trade-Off Values for EQ-5D Health States: Modeling with Observed Values for 101 Health States. *Value Health* **2009**, *12*, 1187–1193. [CrossRef]
24. Yao, Q.; Liu, C.; Zhang, Y. Changes in health-related quality of life of Chinese populations measured by the EQ-5D-3 L: A comparison of the 2008 and 2013 National Health Services Surveys. *Health Qual. Life Outcomes* **2019**, *17*, 1–12. [CrossRef]
25. Kim, K.H.; Lee, S.G. Effects of Health Status and Health Behaviors on Health-related Quality of Life in Korean Adults. *Korean J. Health Serv. Manag.* **2020**, *14*, 161–176. [CrossRef]

26. Bang, S.Y.; Do, Y.S. Health-related Quality of Life of Physical and Mental Health in Middle-aged Women. *J. Korea Acad.-Ind. Coop. Soc.* **2020**, *21*, 161–169. [CrossRef]
27. Yun, H.S. Convergence analysis on the effects of smoking and drinking on quality of life in Adults. *J. Korea Converg. Soc.* **2021**, *12*, 361–368. [CrossRef]
28. Kim, M.C.; Ahn, C.S.; Kim, Y.S. The Effect of Exercise Program for Falls Prevention on Balance and Quality of Life in the Elderly Women. *J. Korean Soc. Phys. Med.* **2010**, *5*, 245–254.
29. Mollinedo-Cardalda, I.; Rodríguez, A.L.; Ferreira, M.; Cancela-Carral, J.M. Benefits of STRENOLD Program on Health-Related Quality of Life in Adults Aged 60 Years or Older. In Common Sport Study. *Int. J. Environ. Res. Public Health* **2021**, *18*, 3253. [CrossRef]
30. Maranesi, E.; Merlo, A.; Fioretti, S.; Zemp, D.D.; Campanini, I.; Quadri, P. A statistical approach to discriminate between non-fallers, rare fallers and frequent fallers in older adults based on posturographic data. *Clin. Biomech.* **2016**, *32*, 8–13. [CrossRef] [PubMed]
31. Leirós-Rodríguez, R.; Romo-Pérez, V.; García-Soidán, J.L. Validity and reliability of a tool for accelerometric assessment of static balance in women. *Eur. J. Physiother.* **2017**, *19*, 243–248. [CrossRef]

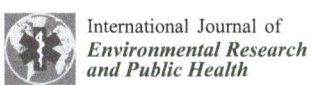

Article

HAPPY MAMA Project (PART 1). Assessing the Reliability of the Italian Karitane Parenting Confidence Scale (KPCS-IT) and Parental Stress Scale (PSS-IT): A Cross-Sectional Study among Mothers Who Gave Birth in the Last 12 Months

Alice Mannocci [1,*], Azzurra Massimi [2], Franca Scaglietta [2], Sara Ciavardini [2], Michela Scollo [2], Claudia Scaglione [2] and Giuseppe La Torre [2]

1. Faculty of Economics, Universitas Mercatorum, 00186 Rome, Italy
2. Department of Public Health and Infectious Diseases, Sapienza University of Rome, 00185 Rome, Italy; azzurra.massimi@uniroma1.it (A.M.); f.scaglietta@gmail.com (F.S.); ciavardini.1695615@studenti.uniroma1.it (S.C.); scollo.1830613@studenti.uniroma1.it (M.S.); scaglione.1634888@studenti.uniroma1.it (C.S.); giuseppe.latorre@uniroma1.it (G.L.T.)
* Correspondence: alice.mannocci@unimercatorum.it

Citation: Mannocci, A.; Massimi, A.; Scaglietta, F.; Ciavardini, S.; Scollo, M.; Scaglione, C.; La Torre, G. HAPPY MAMA Project (PART 1). Assessing the Reliability of the ITalian Karitane Parenting Confidence Scale (KPCS-IT) and Parental Stress Scale (PSS-IT): A Cross-Sectional Study among Mothers Who Gave Birth in the Last 12 Months. *Int. J. Environ. Res. Public Health* **2021**, *18*, 4066. https://doi.org/10.3390/ijerph18084066

Academic Editors: Carmela Mento, Maria Catena Silvestri and Paul Tchounwou

Received: 18 February 2021
Accepted: 8 April 2021
Published: 12 April 2021

Publisher's Note: MDPI stays neutral with regard to jurisdictional claims in published maps and institutional affiliations.

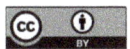

Copyright: © 2021 by the authors. Licensee MDPI, Basel, Switzerland. This article is an open access article distributed under the terms and conditions of the Creative Commons Attribution (CC BY) license (https://creativecommons.org/licenses/by/4.0/).

Abstract: The purposes of this study were: (1) to adapt two validated questionnaires used to evaluate maternal confidence (KPCS-IT) and maternal stress (PSS-IT) to the Italian context, in order to (2) measure the stress level and the self-efficacy in an Italian sample of mothers. The validation process has provided the construction of an online questionnaire. It was administered on a convenience mothers sample with at least a child aged 0–12 months, twice (T0 and T1) with a two day interval. Assessment of instrument stability over time was estimated by applying test–retest reliability between T0 and T1, and the Cronbach's alpha coefficient. A cross-sectional study was carried out to assess the second aim. Italian mothers with at least one child living at home aged between 0–12 months were recruited. Statistical reliability methods were applied to assess the internal validity of the two questionnaires. PSS-IT was analyzed using univariate and multivariate statistical analyses in order to study the association between KPCS-IT, demographic and maternal characteristics. Statistical significance was established as $p < 0.05$. The Cronbach's alpha reported a good level of internal consistency of the questionnaires: PSS-IT alpha = 0.862; KPCS-IT alpha = 0.801. 32% of the mothers declared low maternal confidence and the mean value of PSS-IT was 35.4 (SD = 8). The significant inverse correlation was found between the PSS-IT and the KPCS-IT (coeff = −0.353; $p < 0.001$): this means that a high level of perceived self-efficacy reduces the maternal stress level. The study identifies that interventions on maternal confidence can be useful to support mothers in the first months after delivery in order to prevent stress risk: the perceived self-efficacy is as a modifiable factor and the results of the study indicate that it significantly reduces the PSS-IT and EPDS scores. In future, more field trials are necessary in order to assess the realistic and feasible interventions on maternal confidence and competence to prevent maternal distress.

Keywords: distress; self-efficacy; maternal confidence; maternal wellbeing; post-partum

1. Introduction

Post-partum is a challenging period for mothers, characterized by many deep changes and many developmental stages in the family life cycle [1,2]. During a child's first year, mothers often feel overwhelmed by the new situation and need help and support from their partners, their network and health professionals [3]. However, this need for help and guidance is often under-reported, underestimated [4] and usually unmet [5–7].

It is fundamental for health professionals involved in primary care who work to promote well-being among new families (i.e., family health nurses and midwives) to identify mothers with low confidence, low mood and high stress in the post-partum period [8,9]. The mother's well-being, in fact, may impact on the mother–infant relationship and on the infant's future health, especially during the first year [9].

Several studies have identified low maternal confidence [5], symptoms of depression [10] and parental stress [11] as factors negatively related to the well-being and development of the dyads (mother and infant).

However, only a few standardized screening tools have been evaluated in community settings to assess maternal mood, parental stress and maternal confidence [8].

There are tools concerning the measures used in the literature for assessing maternal stress, confidence and depression. They can be categorized according to the age of the baby.

The Parental Stress Scale (PSS), for example, represents a questionnaire published by Berry et al. [12], that aims to measure parental stress in mothers and fathers with 0–12 months babies.

Confidence may be defined as the amount of beliefs or judgments that a parent holds of his/her capabilities to organize and execute a set of tasks related to parenting a child [13]. It was also defined as the Perception of Parental Self-Efficacy (PPSE). In the literature, there are several instruments to measure the PPSE, such as the Karitane Parenting Confidence Scale (KPCS) [14,15], which can be used for parents of infants aged up to 12 months.

The outcome of post-partum depression, unlike others, is widely investigated. The Edinburgh Postnatal Depression Scale (EPDS) is one of the main tools developed to assess maternal mood [16,17] and is actually validated in the Italian context [16,18].

At present, validated screening tools assessing maternal confidence and stress are lacking in the Italian context. Consequently, there are no Italian studies measuring the prevalence of the distress amongst new Italian mothers.

The first objective of this study is to adapt two validated questionnaires used to evaluate maternal confidence (Karitane Parenting Confidence Scale ITalian version, KPCS-IT) and maternal stress (Parental Stress Scale ITalian version, PSS-IT) to the Italian context, and to evaluate their reliability, their stability over time and their internal consistency [19].

The second and main aim of the study is to measure the stress level, the self-efficacy and the depression risk in an Italian sample of mothers with at least one child under the age of 12 months.

2. Material and Methods

The present study was divided in two main sections: the validation of the instruments and a cross-sectional study (the "HAPPY MAMA web survey").

The University Sapienza of Rome Ethics Committees approved the study (protocol number 826/19RIF.CE: 5559).

2.1. Sample

Mothers with at least a child aged 0–12 months were involved in the validation study and in the web-survey.

2.2. Validation of the Instruments

An online questionnaire was used to measure (a) the stress level, (b) self-confidence and (c) risk of depression.

The first two outcomes, a–b, were measured creating an Italian version of the KPCS (KPCS-IT) and PSS (PSS-IT). The risk of depression was measured using the Italian version of EPDS validated by Benvenuti et al. [18].

The questionnaires were chosen on the basis of a search on PubMed using the following search algorithm: self-efficacy OR confidence OR stress OR depression AND (mother OR new–mother OR parental) AND (questionnaire OR tool OR score OR scale OR measure). The questionnaires founded were be evaluated in a consensus meeting. It involved the Happy MAMA research group with two psychology and cognitive science experts.

The KPCS [14] is a tool designed to assess the perceived parental self-efficacy defined as "beliefs or judgment a parent holds of their capabilities to organize and execute asset of tasks related to parenting a child" [13]. The 15-item scale grounded in the self-efficacy theory [20] returns a score that ranges from 0 to 45. The cut-off score for KPCS was determined according to the Črnčec et al. [14]: parents scoring ≤39 be experiencing low levels of parenting confidence. The transformation of continuous variable to a binary outcome was applied [14].

The PSS is an 18-item questionnaire, and each item is rated on a scale from 1 to 5 [12]. The PSS final score ranged from 18 to 90: a higher score indicates high level of parental stress. A clinical cut-off point for the PSS was not recommended [12].

The EPDS is a self-report screening measure to detect symptoms of postpartum depression. It is a 10-item questionnaire where each item is rated on a scale from 0 to 3 [21]. The clinical cut-off points in different language versions of the EPDS range from 7 to 14 [22]. Internationally the most commonly used clinical cut-off is an EPDS score ≥12: scores >12 on the EPDS are correlated with a diagnosis of major risk of depressive disorder (MDD) [23]. The transformation of continuous outcome to a binary outcome was applied [23].

The PSS-IT and KPCS-IT validations have foreseen the following activities [24]:

a. three independent researchers translated the English version of KPCS and PSS in Italian language, and then a consensus version was realized;
b. the draft of the Italian version was back-translated in English by an interpreter in order to estimate the compliance with the original version and subsequently it was reviewed according to the translation;
c. a telephone survey was conducted on an opportunistic sample of 30 mothers with at least a child aged 0–12 months. It was carried-out in order to obtain feedback on the level of the items comprehension;
d. a second phone survey was conducted in order to assess the stability and to verify the level of comprehension of the new "final" version: the tool was administered twice over a period of two days to the same group of individuals;
e. the final version was transformed in an online questionnaire using Google Form. A convenience mothers sample (called "validation sample") with at least a child aged 0–12 months was involved to complete the same questionnaire twice (T0 and T1) with a two day interval (a "Whatsapp" message or an e-mail containing the link to the questionnaire were used as a reminder). Informative notes, aims and details of the study were reported at the beginning of the questionnaire.

These final versions were called PSS-IT and KPCS-IT.

2.3. HAPPY MAMA Web Survey

2.3.1. Design

The Strengthening the Reporting of Observational Studies in Epidemiology (STROBE) statement for cross-sectional study was followed to perform the HAPPY MAMA web survey [25,26].

2.3.2. Measures

A questionnaire including the PSS-IT, the KPCT-IT, the EPDS and a section with demographic variables (age, civil status, number of sons, region, city, date of the birth, occupation, vaginal or cesarean delivery) were used for data collection of the second aim of the study: "HAPPY MAMA web survey".

The data collection phase was performed in May–June 2019.

2.3.3. Data Collection Strategy

The dissemination of the questionnaire link was made through Facebook groups. Italian Facebook groups with a topic on mother, newborn, pregnancy and post-partum were selected. The link was advertised at least once a week during 40 days.

The "HAPPY MAMA project" Facebook page was created and the questionnaire link was posted.

2.4. Statistical Analysis

The statistical analysis presented in this paragraph was divided in two sections: one dedicated to the validation of the instruments and the second one to the HAPPY MAMA web-based survey. The validation of the instruments includes a reliability analysis. It was applied on PSS-IT KPCS-IT questionnaires.

The following aspects were considered:

1. Assessing of instrument stability over time: test-retest reliability was estimated between T0 and T1, it was calculated with Intra-class Correlation Coefficient (ICC) with absolute agreement and two-way mixed model. The ICC was estimated using the data of "validation sample". Test-retest reliability coefficients vary between 0 and 1 and the interpretation by Streiner et al. [27] was considered:

   - 1: perfect reliability;
   - ≥ 0.9: excellent reliability;
   - $\geq 0.8 < 0.9$: good reliability;
   - $\geq 0.7 < 0.8$: acceptable reliability;
   - $\geq 0.6 < 0.7$: questionable reliability;
   - $\geq 0.5 < 0.6$: poor reliability;
   - < 0.5: unacceptable reliability;
   - 0: no reliability.

2. Correlation: Spearman's coefficient was computed between T0 and T1 of PSS-IT e KPCS-IT scores considering the "validation sample".

3. Assessing internal consistency: Cronbach's alpha coefficient of each questionnaire was applied using a random selection of a sub-group from the sample of the web-survey.

The analysis of the HAPPY MAMA web-based survey included a descriptive, univariate, bivariate and multivariate analysis.

The outcomes considered in the HAPPY MAMA web-based survey were the score obtained by PSS-IT and Benvenuti's EPDS version [18]. The KPCS-IT score was used as a dependent variable and risk factor.

The descriptive statistics of background variables and outcomes were realized using means, SDs for continuous variables and frequencies with percentages for qualitative ones.

The univariate analysis was realized in order to assess the possible association with PSS-IT versus age, having sons, delivery characteristics, months after delivery and KPCS and EPDS scores. The central limit theorem ensures that parametric tests can be used with large samples (n > 30), even if the hypotheses of normality are violated [28,29]. Therefore, the T-Student and ANOVA parametric tests were used for the comparison of parental stress between groups of subjects.

ANOVA with a post-hoc Bonferroni test was used to determine the differences among the four quarters (Months after delivery).

The Pearson's correlation coefficients (r) were calculated to investigate how strongly the three measurements (KPCS-IT, EPDS and PSS-IT) were internally related.

To determine predictors of the PSS-IT score a multivariate linear regression model was performed. The inclusion of any covariate in the model was decided on the basis of the univariate analysis (p value ≤ 0.25). The fit of the data into the model was tested using the R^2.

Stepwise with backward elimination of non-significant variables (probability to entry $p < 0.05$) was subsequently used to generate a minimal model.

The level of significance was set at $p < 0.05$ for all analysis.

Statistical analysis was performed using the Statistical Package for Social Sciences (SPSS version 25, IBM Corporation, Armonk, NY, USA).

3. Results

3.1. Validation of the Instruments

The phone survey used to perform the Italian translation was conducted on 29 mothers (see point "d" of "Validation of the instruments" in the previous subparagraph). Among those 26 filled out the questionnaire twice and reported the comprehensibility problems of the items.

The "validation sample" included 25 women, of which 22 filled out the questionnaire twice (see point "e" of "Validation of the instruments" in the previous subparagraph).

3.1.1. Translation and Level of the Items Comprehension

The first phone survey for the feedback on the level of the questions comprehension, showed the need of changes in some items (Supplementary File, Table S1):

1. In the KPCS questionnaire followed items were reviews:
   - item 1: "I am confident about feeding my baby . . . " literally translated into Italian "mi sento fiduciosa quando nutro il mio bambino . . . " it was then translated into "Mi sento serena quando do da mangiare al mio bambino" with a more familiar tone;
   - item 3: "I am confident about helping my baby to establish a good sleep routine" literally translated into Italian "Mi sento fiduciosa di aiutare il mio bambino a stabilire un buon ritmo del sonno" it was then translated into "Mi sento in grado di aiutare il mio bambino a stabilire un buon ritmo del sonno" with a more familiar tone;
   - item 7: "I am confident about playing with my baby" literally translated into Italian "Mi sento fiduciosa quando gioco con il mio bambino", it was then translated into "Mi sento tranquilla quando gioco con il mio bambino" with a more familiar tone;
2. In the PSS questionnaire:
   - item 4: "I sometimes worry whether I am doing enough for my child/ren", literally translated into Italian "A volte mi preoccupo se sto facendo abbastanza per mio/miei figlio/i" was then translated into "Mi capita di preoccuparmi di non riuscire a fare abbastanza per mio/miei figlio/i" with a more familiar tone.

3.1.2. Reliability of the Instruments

The second phone survey was given to the "validation sample" and it permitted a test-retest analysis. The ICC was 0.957 between T0 and T1 for PSS-IT score and 0.999 T1 for KPCT-IT. Both coefficients indicated excellent agreement between the measures over time.

Furthermore, the Spearman's coefficient for PSS-IT between T0 and T1 is $r = 0.839$, $p < 0.001$, and for KPCS-IT is $r = 0.999$, $p < 0.001$.

The Cronbach's alpha reported a good level of internal consistency for both PSS-IT (alpha = 0.862) and KPCS-IT (alpha = 0.801). The variation of the alpha value is shown in Table 1 if one item is deleted from the questionnaire. The alpha value was not increased by the removal of items in both questionnaires, except for item 2 and 4 in PSS-IT, but the increase was lower than 0.01.

3.2. Web Survey Analysis: Descriptive, Univariate and Bivariate Analysis

The HAPPY MAMA web survey involved 49 Facebook groups, of which 36 published the questionnaire link (Annex S1, see Supplementary Files). One-thousand and eighty-seven questionnaires were collected. Eight-hundred and seventy-six were valid, the remaining 211 came from pregnant women or mothers with children out of target age. The mean age of women involved in the web survey was 33.8 with SD = 4.5 years. Thirty-one percent of births occur by C-section. Ninety-eight percent had an occupation. The geographical distribution of the mothers was: 28% in the Norther Regions, 47% in the Central and 25% in Southern.

Table 1. Cronbach's alpha of KPCS-IT, PSS-IT scores.

Questionnaire	Item	Cronbach's Alpha if Item Deleted
PSS-IT	1	0.850
	2	**0.863**
	3	0.859
	4	**0.863**
	5	0.857
	6	0.856
	7	0.861
	8	0.857
	9	0.852
	10	0.853
	11	0.858
	12	0.851
	13	0.855
	14	0.856
	15	0.847
	16	0.849
	17	0.852
	18	0.859
	Pooled Cronbach's alpha	**0.862**
KPCS-IT	1	0.792
	2	0.786
	3	0.793
	4	0.783
	5	0.787
	6	0.787
	7	0.787
	8	0.792
	9	0.805
	10	0.783
	11	0.783
	12	0.791
	13	0.781
	14	0.791
	15	0.810
	Pooled Cronbach's alpha	**0.801**

The description of the dichotomized and continuous scores of the KPCS-IT and EPDS (according to the categorization cited in "Material and Methods") are presented in Table 2. The mean values of the scores were: PSS-IT 35.4 (SD = 8.9, CI95%:34.7–36.1); KPCS-IT 36.8 (SD = 5.0, CI95%:36.4–37.2) and EPDS 9.7 (SD = 5.2, CI95%:9.3–10.0).

Table 2. Descriptive statistics of HAPPY MAMA web-based survey' sample.

Variables			
Qualitative		n	%
Cesarean delivery	No	270	69
	Yes	606	31
Gestational age (weeks)	≥38	782	89
	<38	94	11
Lives with infant's father	Yes	856	98
	No	12	1
	No answer	8	1

Table 2. Cont.

Variables			
Qualitative		n	%
Geographical area where she lives	North	248	28
	Center	410	47
	South	218	25
Months after delivery (quarters)	1st	192	22
	2nd	251	29
	3rd	191	22
	4th	242	27
Number of sons	1	572	65
	>1	304	35
Age groups (years)	≤31	269	32
	32–35	281	32
	≥36	296	34
Employed/student or housewife	Yes	777	89
	No	99	11
KPCS-IT [a] (perception of self-efficacy)	Yes	591	68
	No	283	32
EPDS [a] (presence risk of depression)	Low	603	69
	High	273	31
Quantitative		Mean	SD
PSS-IT score		35.4	8.9
KPCS-IT score		36.8	5.0
EPDS score		9.7	5.2

[a] Dichotomous variable. The cut-off point is defined according to the literature (see "Material and Methods" paragraph).

The univariate analysis was shown in Table 3. There were significant associations between the high PSS-IT score and working women ($p = 0.016$), time elapsed after the delivery ($p = 0.006$), women with two or more children ($p < 0.001$), women with a low level of parenting confidence ($p < 0.001$) and women with a high risk of depression ($p < 0.001$).

Table 3. Univariate analysis of PSS-IT score versus the variables studied.

Variables		PSS-IT Score			Test
		Mean	SD	p	
Cesarean delivery	Yes	35.62	9.04	0.774	T-student
	No	35.44	8.96		
Gestational age (weeks)	≥38	35.2	8.2	0.688	T-student
	<38	35.5	9.2		
Employed	Yes	35.2	8.8	0.016	T-student
	No	37.5	9.6		
Geographical area where she lives	North	35.57	8.45	0.358	Anova
	Center	35.09	9.26		
	South	36.16	9.01		
Months after delivery (quarters)	1st	34.84	8.52	0.006 *	ANOVA *
	2nd	34.59	8.81		
	3rd	35.18	8.96		
	4th	37.20	9.33		
Number of sons	1	34.71	9.16	<0.001	T-student
	>1	36.97	8.44		

Table 3. Cont.

Variables		PSS-IT Score			Test
		Mean	SD	p	
Age groups (years)	≤31	34.71	8.97	0.178	Anova
	32–35	35.82	8.97		
	≥36	36.01	8.84		
KPCS-IT [a]	Yes	30.05	6.58	<0.001	Anova
	No	38.13	8.8		
EPDS [a]	Low	32.45	6.95	<0.001	Anova
	High	42.22	9.30		

Bold: The mean difference is significant at the <0.05 level. a. Dichotomous variable. The cut-off point is defined according to the literature (see "Material and Methods" paragraph). * The Bonferroni's post-hoc analysis to assess the difference between the quarters (p-value was set at $p < 0.05/4 = 0.0125$).

(I) Quarter	(J) Quarter	Mean Difference (I–J)	Bonferroni's Test p Value	95% CI	
				Lower	Upper
1	2	0.25	0.99	−2.01	2.51
	3	−0.33	0.99	−2.75	2.08
	4	−2.35	0.04	−4.64	−0.07
2	1	−0.25	0.99	−2.51	2.01
	3	−0.58	0.99	−2.85	1.68
	4	−2.60	**0.01**	**−4.73**	**−0.48**
3	1	0.33	0.99	−2.08	2.75
	2	0.58	0.99	−1.68	2.85
	4	−2.02	0.12	−4.31	0.26
4	1	2.35	0.04	0.07	4.64
	2	2.60	**0.01**	**0.48**	**4.73**
	3	2.02	0.12	−0.26	4.31

The Pearson's correlation analysis showed significant direct correlations between the PSS-IT versus EPDS ($r = 0.595$, $p < 0.001$), number of children ($r = 0.08$, $p = 0.40$) and the number of days after the birth ($r = 0.134$, $p < 0.001$). An inverse significant correlation was found with KPCS-IT ($r = -0.577$, $p < 0.001$) as it is illustrated in Figure 1.

Multivariate analysis is reported in Table 4. The findings indicated that the covariates significantly associated to the high PSS-IT level were: days from delivery (coeff = 0.05; $p < 0.001$) and risk of depression (coeff = 0.378; $p < 0.001$); while the covariates significantly associated to the low PSS-IT level were having only one child (coeff = −0.135; $p < 0.001$) and a high self-efficacy score (coeff = −0.353; $p < 0.001$). In the regression model the goodness-of-fit for PSS-IT was $R^2 = 0.455$ (dependent variables explain 45.5% of the variability).

Table 4. Multivariate analysis: linear regression model of PSS-IT score.

Covariates		PSS-IT Score	
		Coefficient	p
Employed	Yes	−0.026	0.320
	No *		
Age (years)		0.050	0.053
Days from delivery		0.095	<0.001
Number of sons	1	−0.135	<0.001
	>1 *		

Table 4. *Cont.*

Covariates	PSS-IT Score	
	Coefficient	p
KPCS-IT score	−0.353	<0.001
EPDS score	0.378	<0.001
Goodness-of-fit: R^2	0.455	

* Reference group Bold: *p*-value < 0.05.

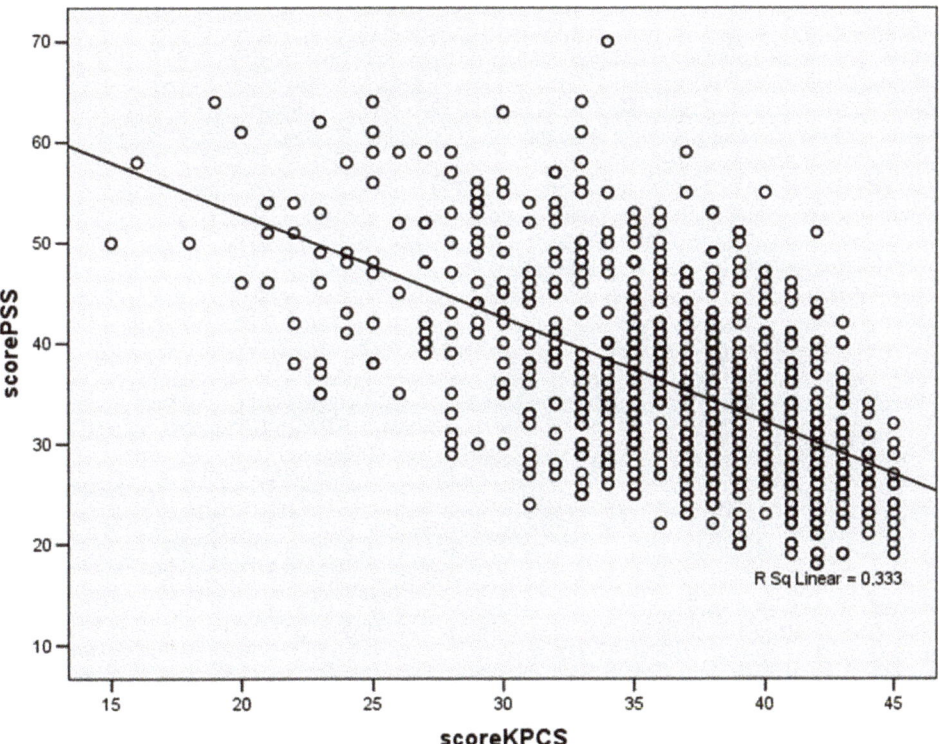

Figure 1. Bivariate analysis: scatter-plot between the PSS-IT and KPC-IT scores.

4. Discussion

The present study supports the validity and the reliability of the PSS-IT and KPCS-IT.

Analyses revealed that the results of both times (T0 and T1) are comparable, thus suggesting the stability of the scale characteristics. Therefore, as parental stress is concerned the PSS-IT has certain advantages: it is easily understandable for mothers and it is brief and easy to administer and score.

According to the literature, the study confirms that the KPCS-IT has easy administration, compilation and scoring [14]. Moreover, the reliability of KPCS-IT and PSS-IT measures of this study are consistent with previous findings: PSS-IT alpha = 0.84% and for KPCS-IT alpha = 0.74% [8].

The second part of the research focused on the cross-sectional study, suggested that the stress level (PSS-IT) is significantly inversely correlated to the self-efficacy (KPCS-IT). This outcome is in agreement with the study's hypothesis. Additionally, a directly significant correlation between the PSS-IT and the EPDS is confirmed.

The correlations of maternal mood, maternal confidence and parental stress are consistent with the previous findings, even when using alternative measures for assessing the parental self-efficacy [8,30]. The obtained mean value of PSS-IT was in agreement with the results of Berry et al. [12] Indeed, their study showed the mean of PSS-IT score in two different groups: in the clinical group it was 43.2 (SD = 9.1; n = 51) and in the control group was 37.1 (n = 116, SD = 8.1; CI95%:35.6–38.6).

Furthermore, the findings of this study underline a gradual significant increase in the parental stress during the 12 month postpartum, and this is in agreement with the results of previous publications [8,31,32].

This study had several limitations. Concerning the first part of the study, "validation and reliability", the test-retest analysis could be not robust, because the guidelines recommended using a sample size as large as possible, but given the variation in the types of used questionnaire, there are no absolute rules for the sample size needed to validate a questionnaire [24]. Moreover, although the sample size was comparable to numerous other test-retest reliability studies [33], small sample sizes have the limit of creating some instability in the alpha coefficients and results must be interpreted with caution.

Concerning the limitations of the second part of the study, a peculiar limitation of the Web survey is due to the cross-sectional design, because the exposure (maternal self-efficacy perception) and outcome (maternal stress level) are simultaneously assessed, there is generally no evidence of a temporal relationship between exposure and outcome.

Secondly, the external validity of the study may be affected by the exclusive presence of Facebook social network female users. It may have influenced the individual characteristics. It is nonetheless true that female social network users in 2018 represent the 66% of female population between 16–74 of age according to EUROSTAT and ISTAT data [34,35].

Another limit of the web-survey was the low sample size. In Italy, the births are about 435,000 for a year [36]. The size of the sample studied was n = 1087, which means that about 0.25% of the population are new mothers.

A possible selection bias could be included in the results. The women with a premature delivery, or infants with some sequelae after the birth or a major complication in the delivery could have participated more than women with no delivery or infant complications. This aspect could underestimate the stress levels and this could affect the research results.

Furthermore, the study did not take into account if there were external supports such as child-care interventions. This aspect can reduce significantly the stress-level.

Moreover the coefficient of multiple determination for regression model, R^2, indicated that the strength of the relationship between the model and the PSS-IT was low. Approximately half of the observed variation of PSS-IT can be explained by the model's inputs.

5. Conclusions

In conclusion, about one third of the mothers involved in the study declared low maternal confidence and 31% had a high risk of depression. The mean value of parental stress score was in agreement with the literature.

Furthermore, the study identifies potential areas of social support and practice: interventions on maternal confidence may be needed to support mothers in the first months following delivery in order to prevent stress risk: the perceived self-efficacy is a modifiable factor and the results of the present study indicate that it reduces at significant level the parental stress and depression risk. In the future, more research in this area is required and, in particular, more field trials are necessary in order to assess realistic and feasible interventions on maternal confidence and competence to prevent maternal distress.

Supplementary Materials: The following are available online at https://www.mdpi.com/article/10.3390/ijerph18084066/s1, Supplementary File: Annex S1—List of the Facebook groups involved, Table S1: PSS-IT and KPCS-IT Questionnaires.

Author Contributions: A.M. (Alice Mannocci) had the original idea for the paper, which was further developed in discussions with A.M. (Azzurra Massimi) and G.L.T., A.M. (Alice Mannocci) led the statistical analysis. A.M. (Alice Mannocci), A.M. (Azzurra Massimi), S.C., M.S., C.S., led the development of validation of the questionnaires. Research survey. A.M. (Alice Mannocci), A.M. (Azzurra Massimi), F.S. and G.L.T. designed and manage the Research survey in Italy. A.M. (Alice Mannocci), A.M. (Azzurra Massimi), S.C., M.S., C.S., manage the collection of the survey data reported in this study. A.M. (Alice Mannocci) and G.L.T. wrote the first draft of the manuscript. All authors contributed to subsequent drafts and approved the final manuscript. All authors have read and agreed to the published version of the manuscript.

Funding: This research received no external funding.

Institutional Review Board Statement: Not applicable.

Informed Consent Statement: Not applicable

Data Availability Statement: Not applicable.

Acknowledgments: We thank Insa Backhaus, Ornella Di Bella, for their helpful to the earlier drafts of the validated questionnaires. Maria Cristina Di Giovancarlo (Research Center Impresapiens, Sapienza University of Rome) and Tomaso Venditti for their translation support, and all the people who participated in the study.

Conflicts of Interest: The authors declare no conflict of interest.

References

1. Cowan, C.P.; Cowan, P.A. Interventions to Ease the Transition to Parenthood: Why They are Needed and What They Can Do. *Fam. Relat. Interdiscip. J. Appl. Fam. Stud.* **1995**, *44*, 412–423. [CrossRef]
2. Cheng, C.-Y.; Li, Q. Integrative Review of Research on General Health Status and Prevalence of Common Physical Health Conditions of Women after Childbirth. *Women Health Issues* **2008**, *18*, 267–280. [CrossRef] [PubMed]
3. Nyström, K.; Ohrling, K. Parenthood Experiences during the Child's First Year: Literature Review. *J. Adv. Nurs.* **2004**, *46*, 319–330. [CrossRef]
4. Rouhi, M.; Stirling, C.; Ayton, J.; Crisp, E.P. Women's Help-Seeking Behaviours within the First Twelve Months after Childbirth: A Systematic Qualitative Meta-Aggregation Review. *Midwifery* **2019**, *72*, 39–49. [CrossRef] [PubMed]
5. Phelps, J.L.; Belsky, J.; Crnic, K. Earned Security, Daily Stress, and Parenting: A Comparison of Five Alternative Models. *Dev. Psychopathol.* **1998**, *10*, 21–38. [CrossRef]
6. Leahy-Warren, P.; McCarthy, G.; Corcoran, P. First-Time Mothers: Social Support, Maternal Parental Self-Efficacy and Postnatal Depression. *J. Clin. Nurs.* **2012**, *21*, 388–397. [CrossRef] [PubMed]
7. Kronborg, H.; Vaeth, M.; Kristensen, I. The Effect of Early Postpartum Home Visits by Health Visitors: A Natural Experiment. *Public Health Nurs.* **2012**, *29*, 289–301. [CrossRef]
8. Kristensen, I.H.; Simonsen, M.; Trillingsgaard, T.; Pontoppidan, M.; Kronborg, H. First-Time Mothers' Confidence Mood and Stress in the First Months Postpartum. A Cohort Study. *Sex. Reprod. Healthc.* **2018**, *17*, 43–49. [CrossRef]
9. Sroufe, L.A. Attachment and Development: A Prospective, Longitudinal Study from Birth to Adulthood. *Attach. Hum. Dev.* **2005**, *7*, 349–367. [CrossRef]
10. Lilja, G.; Edhborg, M.; Nissen, E. Depressive Mood in Women at Childbirth Predicts Their Mood and Relationship with Infant and Partner during the First Year Postpartum. *Scand. J. Caring Sci.* **2012**, *26*, 245–253. [CrossRef]
11. Jones, T.L.; Prinz, R.J. Potential Roles of Parental Self-Efficacy in Parent and Child Adjustment: A Review. *Clin. Psychol. Rev.* **2005**, *25*, 341–363. [CrossRef]
12. Berry, J.O.; Jones, W.H. The Parental Stress Scale: Initial Psychometric Evidence. *J. Soc. Pers. Relatsh.* **1995**, *12*, 463–472. [CrossRef]
13. Montigny, F.; Lacharité, C. Perceived Parental Efficacy: Concept Analysis. *J. Adv. Nurs.* **2005**, *49*, 387–396. [CrossRef]
14. Crncec, R.; Barnett, B.; Matthey, S. Development of an Instrument to Assess Perceived Self-Efficacy in the Parents of Infants. *Res. Nurs. Health* **2008**, *31*, 442–453. [CrossRef]
15. Crncec, R.; Barnett, B.; Matthey, S. Review of Scales of Parenting Confidence. *J. Nurs. Meas.* **2010**, *18*, 210–240. [CrossRef] [PubMed]
16. Carpiniello, B.; Pariante, C.M.; Serri, F.; Costa, G.; Carta, M.G. Validation of the Edinburgh Postnatal Depression Scale in Italy. *J. Psychosom. Obstet. Gynaecol.* **1997**, *18*, 280–285. [CrossRef] [PubMed]
17. Cox, J.L.; Holden, J.M.; Sagovsky, R. Detection of Postnatal Depression. Development of the 10-Item Edinburgh Postnatal Depression Scale. *Br. J. Psychiatry* **1987**, *150*, 782–786. [CrossRef]
18. Benvenuti, P.; Ferrara, M.; Niccolai, C.; Valoriani, V.; Cox, J.L. The Edinburgh Postnatal Depression Scale: Validation for an Italian Sample. *J. Affect. Disord.* **1999**, *53*, 137–141. [CrossRef]
19. de Vet, H.C.W.; Terwee, C.B.; Mokkink, L.B.; Knol, D.L. *Measurement in Medicine A Practical Guide*; Cambridge University Press: Cambridge, UK, 2011.

20. Bandura, A. Regulation of Cognitive Processes through Perceived Self-Efficacy. *Dev. Psychol.* **1989**, *25*, 729–735. [CrossRef]
21. Cox, R.A.F. *Offshore Medicine Medical Care of Employees in the Offshore Oil Industry*; Springer: London, UK, 1987; ISBN 978-1-4471-1395-9.
22. Zubaran, C.; Schumacher, M.; Roxo, M.R.; Foresti, K. Screening Tools for Postpartum Depression: Validity and Cultural Dimensions. *Afr. J. Psychiatry* **2010**, *13*, 357–365. [CrossRef]
23. Jardri, R.; Pelta, J.; Maron, M.; Thomas, P.; Delion, P.; Codaccioni, X.; Goudemand, M. Predictive Validation Study of the Edinburgh Postnatal Depression Scale in the First Week after Delivery and Risk Analysis for Postnatal Depression. *J. Affect. Disord.* **2006**, *93*, 169–176. [CrossRef]
24. Tsang, S.; Royse, C.; Terkawi, A. Guidelines for Developing, Translating, and Validating a Questionnaire in Perioperative and Pain Medicine. *Saudi J. Anaesth.* **2017**, *11*, 80. [CrossRef]
25. von Elm, E.; Altman, D.G.; Egger, M.; Pocock, S.J.; Gøtzsche, P.C.; Vandenbroucke, J.P. STROBE Initiative Strengthening the Reporting of Observational Studies in Epidemiology (STROBE) Statement: Guidelines for Reporting Observational Studies. *BMJ* **2007**, *335*, 806–808. [CrossRef]
26. von Elm, E.; Altman, D.G.; Egger, M.; Pocock, S.J.; Gøtzsche, P.C.; Vandenbroucke, J.P. STROBE Initiative The Strengthening the Reporting of Observational Studies in Epidemiology (STROBE) Statement: Guidelines for Reporting Observational Studies. *J. Clin. Epidemiol.* **2008**, *61*, 344–349. [CrossRef]
27. Streiner, D.L.; Norman, G.R.; Cairney, J. *Health Measurement Scales: A Practical Guide to Their Development and Use*; Oxford University Press: Oxford, UK, 2015; ISBN 978-0-19-968521-9.
28. Rao, P.V. *Statistical Research Methods in the Life Sciences*; Duxbury Press: Pacific Grove, CA, USA, 1998; ISBN 978-0-534-93141-4.
29. Heeren, T.; D'Agostino, R. Robustness of the Two Independent Samples T-Test When Applied to Ordinal Scaled Data. *Stat. Med.* **1987**, *6*, 79–90. [CrossRef] [PubMed]
30. Fox, C.R.; Gelfand, D.M. Maternal Depressed Mood and Stress as Related to Vigilance, Self-Efficacy and Mother-Child Interactions. *Early Dev. Parent.* **1994**, *3*, 233–243. [CrossRef]
31. Goecke, T.W.; Voigt, F.; Faschingbauer, F.; Spangler, G.; Beckmann, M.W.; Beetz, A. The Association of Prenatal Attachment and Perinatal Factors with Pre- and Postpartum Depression in First-Time Mothers. *Arch. Gynecol. Obstet.* **2012**, *286*, 309–316. [CrossRef]
32. Hsu, H.-C.; Wickrama, K.A.S. Maternal Life Stress and Health during the First 3 Years Postpartum. *Women Health* **2018**, *58*, 565–582. [CrossRef] [PubMed]
33. Green, J.; Young, J.A. Test-Retest Reliability Study of the Barthel Index, the Rivermead Mobility Index, the Nottingham Extended Activities of Daily Living Scale and the Frenchay Activities Index in Stroke Patients. *Disabil. Rehabil.* **2001**, *23*, 670–676. [CrossRef] [PubMed]
34. ISTAT. The Life of Women and Men in Europe-Internet Habits. Available online: https://www.istat.it/donne-uomini/bloc-3c.html?lang=it (accessed on 9 December 2020).
35. EUROSTAT Individuals—Frequency of Internet Use. Available online: http://appsso.eurostat.ec.europa.eu/nui/show.do?query=BOOKMARK_DS-053748_QID_7B4F68C8_UID_-3F171EB0&layout=IND_TYPE,L,X,0;GEO,L,Y,0;INDIC_IS,L,Z,0;UNIT,L,Z,1;TIME,C,Z,2;INDICATORS,C,Z,3;&zSelection=DS-053748TIME,2016;DS-053748UNIT,PC_IND;DS-053748INDICATORS,OBS_FLAG;DS-053748INDIC_IS,I_IUSE;&rankName1=UNIT_1_2_-1_2&rankName2=INDICATORS_1_2_-1_2&rankName3=INDIC-IS_1_2_-1_2&rankName4=TIME_1_0_1_0&rankName5=IND-TYPE_1_2_0_0&rankName6=GEO_1_2_0_1&rStp=&cStp=&rDCh=&cDCh=&rDM=true&cDM=true&footnes=false&empty=false&wai=false&time_mode=NONE&time_most_recent=false&lang=EN&cfo=%23%23%23%2C%23%23%23.%23%23%23&lang=it (accessed on 4 December 2020).
36. Italian Minister of Health. Direzione Generale della Digitalizzazione del Sistema Informativo Sanitario e della Statistica. In *Ufficio di Statistica Certificato Di Assistenza al Parto (CeDAP)Analisi Dell'evento Nascita-Anno 2018*; Attività Editoriali Ministero della Salute, Italy; 2018. Available online: http://www.salute.gov.it/imgs/C_17_pubblicazioni_3034_allegato.pdf (accessed on 4 April 2021).

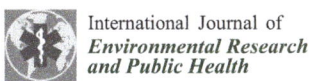

Article

Analysis of Effectiveness of Individual and Group Trauma-Focused Interventions for Female Victims of Intimate Partner Violence

María Crespo *, María Arinero and Carmen Soberón

Department Personality, Assessment and Clinical Psychology, Universidad Complutense de Madrid, 28223 Madrid, Spain; arinerom@yahoo.es (M.A.); c.soberon@ucm.es (C.S.)
* Correspondence: mcrespo@psi.ucm.es; Tel.: +34-913-942-831

Abstract: Group psychological programs for intimate partner violence (IPV) survivors would seem particularly useful since they contribute to interrupting women's isolation and have cost-effectiveness advantage. This study aims to analyze whether the effectiveness of group interventions for female survivors of IPV is equivalent to that of the individual format. A cognitive-behavioral trauma-focused intervention program was applied in eight weekly sessions in Madrid (Spain) to IPV female survivors with significant posttraumatic symptoms that were randomly assigned to the individual ($n = 25$) or group ($n = 28$) intervention format. Measures of posttraumatic stress (Severity of Posttraumatic Stress Disorder Symptoms Scale), depression (Beck Depression Inventory), anxiety (Beck Anxiety Inventory), self-esteem (Rosenberg's Scale) and social support were analyzed at pre-treatment, post-treatment, and 1-, 3-, 6- and 12-months follow-ups. A total of 28.3% of women dropped out, without significant format differences. Intervention (both formats) had significant improvements with large effect sizes in posttraumatic stress ($\eta^2_p = 0.56$), depression ($\eta^2_p = 0.45$), anxiety ($\eta^2_p = 0.41$) and self-esteem ($\eta^2_p = 0.26$) that maintained in follow-ups ($p < 0.001$), without significant differences between formats. Both intervention formats had different evolutions for depression and anxiety ($p < 0.05$), with better effects in the individual format at the first post-test measurements, but the differences tended to disappear over time. Intervention was effective in improving social support, with no significant differences between formats. All in all, both formats showed similar effectiveness. The group format could be an alternative when applying psychological interventions for female IPV survivors, since it would maintain good cost-effectiveness balance, mainly in the long-term.

Keywords: intimate partner violence; psychological treatment; randomized controlled trial; posttraumatic stress; effectiveness

Citation: Crespo, M.; Arinero, M.; Soberón, C. Analysis of Effectiveness of Individual and Group Trauma-Focused Interventions for Female Victims of Intimate Partner Violence. *Int. J. Environ. Res. Public Health* **2021**, *18*, 1952. https://doi.org/10.3390/ijerph18041952

Academic Editor: Maria Catena Silvestri

Received: 10 December 2020
Accepted: 13 February 2021
Published: 17 February 2021

Publisher's Note: MDPI stays neutral with regard to jurisdictional claims in published maps and institutional affiliations.

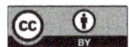

Copyright: © 2021 by the authors. Licensee MDPI, Basel, Switzerland. This article is an open access article distributed under the terms and conditions of the Creative Commons Attribution (CC BY) license (https://creativecommons.org/licenses/by/4.0/).

1. Introduction

Intimate partner violence (IPV) is currently one of the major public health problems around the world; according to the systematic review on violence against women published by the World Health Organization [1], the global prevalence of physical and/or sexual intimate partner violence among all ever-partnered women was 30.0%. Similarly, data from the nationally representative Spanish Survey on Violence Against Women 2015 suggest that 30.7% of Spanish women aged 16 and above have experienced at least one type of IPV during their lives, and 13.2% reported IPV in the 12 months prior to the assessment [2], while according to the 2015 National Intimate Partner and Sexual Violence Survey, 33.6% of women in the United States have experienced rape, physical violence, and/or stalking by an intimate partner in their lifetime, and 5.2% in the last 12-months [3].

Women victims of IPV are exposed to chronic and often extreme maltreatment that can lead to a broad range of physical, social and psychological outcomes. In their systematic review, Langdon et al. [4] concluded that IPV can have more adverse effects on mental health in comparison to non-IPV victims and victims of other traumatic events, being Posttraumatic Stress Disorder (PTSD), depression and anxiety, which are the most consistent mental health outcomes associated with IPV across the studies. Actually, the recent WHO World Mental Health Survey [5] posed the physical abuse by a partner as one of the traumatic events that conveys the greatest risk for PTSD. Likewise, IPV has also been associated with other relevant variables, such as suicidal ideation [6,7], alcohol and substances use [8], poor health status and self-perceived health [2,6], somatization [4], and functional impairments [9].

On the basis of increasing rates of IPV and its potential consequences, in the last twenty years, a considerable number of interventions have been designed or modified specifically for IPV survivors. In a systematic review and meta-analysis about short-term interventions for survivors of IPV, Arroyo et al. [10] found that most interventions analyzed were effective compared to not receiving treatment, achieving large effect sizes in PTSD, self-esteem, depression, general distress and life functioning. Regarding treatment type, largest effects sizes were found for cognitive behavioral therapies (CBT) and interpersonal therapies specifically tailored to IPV survivors. In addition, individually delivered interventions produced significantly stronger outcomes than group delivered interventions. However, authors noted that some methodological weaknesses in analyzed studies could have biased their findings.

Individual interventions may lead to a closer attention to survivors, and therefore could be more tailored and targeted to the specific needs of women [10]. In addition, some IPV survivors could prefer individual interventions because they may feel worse sharing their problems in a therapeutic group [11]. Furthermore, the implementation of some intervention techniques, such as exposure therapy, could be more problematic in the group delivery format [12]. However, regarding cost-effectiveness, it may be difficult to deliver individual interventions in settings where economic and human sources are limited [13]. Likewise, group interventions may convey additional benefits to women victims of IPV from a social perspective; the group could be a source of social learning where IPV survivors could change and acquire skills through interactions with other women facing similar situations [13,14]; additionally, the group may also provide social support [13,14], a relevant protective factor against IPV mental health outcomes [6]. In this sense group programs would be adequate to interrupt women's isolation and would seem particularly useful for long term or chronic posttraumatic symptoms [15]. Furthermore, the group format is often chosen for delivering interventions due to its cost-effectiveness advantage [15].

Despite the clinical relevance of the intervention delivery type, the only study that has directly compared the effectiveness of an intervention program tailored to female IPV survivors in the individual versus group format was by Fernández-Velasco's [12]. In this study, which included 95 Spanish women victims of IPV, both intervention delivery types have proven to be effective to treat PTSD, depression, self-esteem and general maladjustment, although the individual format was superior to group intervention, mainly at 6- and 12-months follow-ups. However, as the author noted, the fact that two different therapists implemented each intervention format could have skewed these findings. In addition, this study only includes IPV survivors who met the criteria for PTSD diagnosis, which may limit the generalizability of these findings to IPV victims who may manifest sub-clinical levels of posttraumatic symptoms that are nonetheless seriously disabling and may require psychological intervention. Finally, regarding social variables, although this study included a measure of maladjustment associated with overall symptomatology, it did not specifically associate this impairment to posttraumatic symptoms, and it did not assess other important social variables in IPV survivors such as social support.

The purpose of the present study was to explore the differential effectiveness of individual and group intervention for female survivors of IPV. Therefore, it involves a comparison of individual vs. group formats of a brief CBT trauma-focused intervention program that has previously showed its effectiveness for women victims of IPV with sub-clinical PTSD symptoms (cf. [16]).

2. Materials and Methods

2.1. Objectives and Hypotheses

To establish the differential effectiveness of the individual and group delivery formats, the study analyzes format differences in adherence to treatment, as well as efficacy and clinical significance of the improvements achieved in the posttreatment and at 1-, 3-, 6- and 12 months follow-ups. Primary outcome variables were overall posttraumatic symptoms, and associated symptoms of depression and anxiety. Other variables relevant to battered women emotional status (namely self-esteem) were considered to be secondary variables. Moreover, in order to assess the specific effects of both formats on social issues, we also examined variables such as social and family support.

Based on previous research, it was hypothesized that (1) adherence to treatment would be higher in the individual format than in the group one; (2) both intervention formats would reduce posttraumatic symptoms, depression and anxiety, and increase self-esteem, and would produce clinically significant changes; (3) individual format effect on outcome variables would be superior; and (4) group format would show a higher effect on social issues.

2.2. Participants

Participants were recruited from several organizations and institutions in the area of Madrid (Spain), which offered programs for women that suffer IPV. All the women that initially attended these services for attention because of IPV were assessed to establish the eligibility criteria: being woman 18 years of age or older, having suffered violence by a male intimate partner, presenting posttraumatic symptoms in the Severity of Posttraumatic Stress Disorder Symptoms Scale [17] without meeting all the diagnostic criteria for PTSD according to the Diagnostic and Statistical Manual of Mental Disorders, 4th ed. revised [18]; and receiving no other current treatment. When a woman presented symptoms that met all the diagnostic criteria for PTSD, she was derived to a parallel treatment specifically designed for battered women with PTSD that was carried out by a different research team. Exclusion criteria included conditions that could prevent compliance with the treatment (namely, abuse of alcohol or drugs, cognitive impairment or illiteracy in Spanish).

One-hundred and sixteen women were initially assessed. Nineteen were excluded for meeting PTSD diagnostic criteria and 19 rejected the treatment for different reasons (schedule problems, change of residence, etc.). Consequently, 78 accepted the treatment; nevertheless, this study reports the data of 53, since the other 25 were included in a former phase of the project [16]. Their participation in the treatment was voluntary and was always carried out after the women were informed of the goal of the study and guaranteeing the confidentiality of the information provided. Figure 1 illustrates the participants CONSORT (Consolidated Standards of Reporting Trials) diagram.

2.3. Design

A multigroup (two groups) experimental design was employed with repeated pre- and post-measures (2 months later) and follow-up measures taken at 1, 3, 6 and 12 months after the end of the treatment. The independent variable was the psychological intervention (a brief multicomponent CBT program), with two levels according to their delivering format: individual vs. group.

Participants were assigned to each experimental condition by a balanced random process using the randomization.com computer program (cf. http://www.randomization.com (accessed on 10 December 2020)). In this way, 28 participants were assigned to the group format and 25 to the individual one. The study protocol was approved by the Faculty Ethics Committee (number 2016/17-022) and it was conducted following CONSORT recommendations [19].

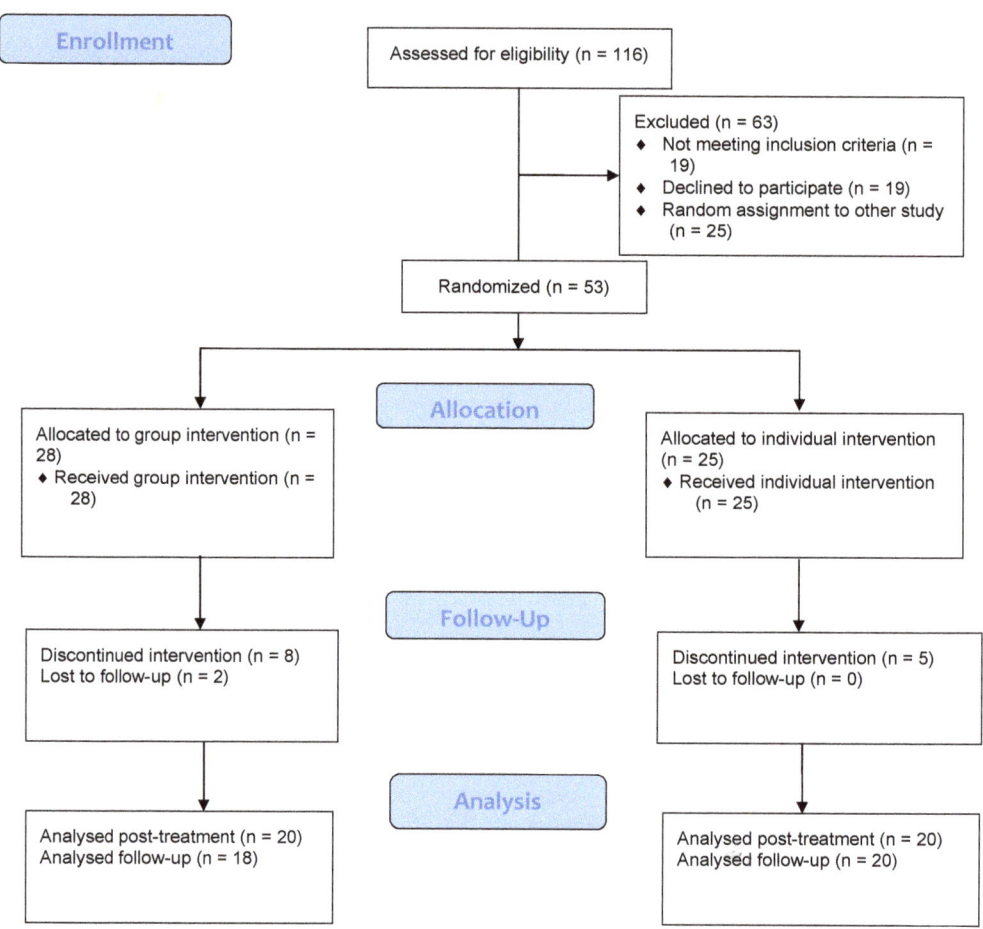

Figure 1. CONSORT participants flow diagram.

2.4. Variables and Measures

2.4.1. Demographic Variables and History and Features of Violence

A standardized interview [20] assessed background information (e.g., age, subjective social class, educational level, civil status, etc.), and information about the history and features of violence, considering the type, duration, frequency, need of help and attention (legal, medical and psychiatric/psychological), and perception of support received (familiar and social). The interview included the Cut-down, Annoyed, Guilty and Eye-opener-CAGE questionnaire ([21]; Spanish translation by Fonseca del Pozo et al. [22]) to assess the possibility of abusive consumption of alcohol. In Spanish samples, the CAGE has shown a sensitivity of 96% and a specificity of 100% at a cutoff point of 1 [23].

2.4.2. Outcome Variables

Severity of Posttraumatic Stress Disorder Symptoms Scale (in Spanish Escala de Gravedad de Síntomas del Trastorno de Estrés Postraumático, EGS; Echeburúa et al. [17]) was used to assess the severity of posttraumatic symptoms ranging from 0 to 51 (higher scores showing more severe symptoms). The test-retest reliability coefficient of this scale was 0.89 ($p \leq 0.001$) with a 4-week interval, and its internal consistency index (Cronbach's alpha) was 0.92. The global score reaches a sensitivity of 100% and a specificity of 93.7% at a cut-off point of 15 to 16.

Beck Depression Inventory (BDI-II; Beck et al. [24], in the Spanish version by Sanz et al. [25]) identifies the global level of depression and the changes over time. The scores range was 0–63 (higher scores showing more severe symptoms). The published Spanish adaptation of the BDI-II [25] proposes a cut-off point of 13 to differentiate the minimum or slight levels of depression from moderate or severe levels. The Spanish version of the inventory has shown good internal consistency: 0.90 with subclinical samples [26] and 0.89 with patients presenting diverse disorders [27].

Beck Anxiety Inventory (BAI; Beck et al. [28], in the Spanish version by Sanz and Navarro [29]) assesses anxiety symptoms, focusing particularly on the physiological symptoms (66.7%). The remaining items refer to affective (14.3%) and cognitive aspects (19%). The scores range was 0–63 (higher scores showing more severe symptoms). According to Sanz [30], a cut-off point of 13 differentiates normal or slight levels of anxiety from moderate to severe levels. The internal consistency of the Spanish version was satisfactory ($\alpha = 0.88$).

Rosenberg's Self-Esteem Scale (Rosenberg [31]; Spanish version by Echeburúa and Corral [32]) assesses women's levels of self-esteem, which is a person's feelings of self-satisfaction and self-acceptance. The scores range was 10–40 (higher scores showing higher self-esteem) and a cut-off point of 29 differentiates low from high self-esteem. Its internal consistency was 0.81 and its discriminant validity was adequate.

All these instruments, except the standardized interview that was applied only in pre-treatment assessment, were readministered at post-treatment and the follow-ups. Additionally, the Client Satisfaction Questionnaire (CSQ-8; Larsen et al. [33]; Spanish version by Echeburúa and Corral [32]) was introduced in post-treatment assessment to evaluate the quality of the program and the women's satisfaction with the treatment. The scores range was 8–32, showing higher scores greater satisfaction.

2.5. Procedure

The treatment used in this study was a multicomponent cognitive-behavioral program based on Rincón and Labrador's work [20] that, on the basis of the specific needs of this population and through a review of prior treatment studies, includes the following modules: (a) psycho-education, providing the participants information about IPV and its consequences for the victim; (b) exercises to control arousal by diaphragmatic breathing (focused on hyper-alertness symptoms); (c) planning to increase pleasant activities as a way to improve mood; (d) specific techniques to improve self-esteem; (e) restructuring of biased cognitions; (f) increase of skills for an independent life (by training in problem-solving); (g) exposure techniques in imagination focused on the memory of IPV situations to address re-experiencing and avoidance responses; and (h) relapse prevention.

All in all, the program consisted of 8 weekly sessions (which implies a total program duration of two months). The first session included presentations and the establishment of the treatment rules besides some information about the violence and about the intervention format. The other sessions started with a brief "check in" and review of the homework, followed by some new elements (cognitive-behavioral skills) to discuss and practice, and ended with 5 min of diaphragmatic breathing. The specific content for each session was as follows: (1) psycho-education (session 1); (2) exercises of diaphragmatic breathing (sessions 1–7); (3) planning to increase pleasant activities (sessions 2–3); (4) techniques to improve self-esteem (sessions 2–3); (5) cognitive restructuring of biased cognitions (sessions 2–4); (6) training in problem-solving (sessions 4–5); and (7) exposure techniques (sessions 6–7). Finally, session 8 was focused on relapse prevention.

Sessions lasted 60 min for the individual format and 90 min for the group version. Group format intervention was delivered in groups of 3–5 women. Between sessions, the women of both experimental groups received written material that outlined the topics from the session, as well as exercises to be done as homework. Women's performance of trained skills was monitored by counting the number of completed homework sheets returned by each woman over the duration of the study. Assessment was performed individually before treatment and then after treatment and the four follow-ups in sessions of about 90 min carried out by the same person.

In order to avoid potential bias, both intervention formats were conducted by the same therapist. Likewise, the intervention protocol and homework sheets were manualized to ensure the homogeneity and replicability. Further details about the program can be found elsewhere [16,34]. The manual of the intervention protocol as well as all the therapeutic materials are available upon request to the authors.

2.6. Data Analysis

Analyses were performed using an intent-to-treat (ITT) approach. Little's MCAR test [35] showed that the data were missing completely at random (MCAR), so that the maximum likelihood estimation was applied for replacement. Kolmogorov-Smirnov tests and Levene's test for equality of variances were applied to check the distribution of the data for the pretreatment measure of the outcome variables in the two experimental conditions. Since the results confirmed normal distribution and equality of variances, independent samples t-test, Chi-square test and Fisher exact test were used to verify the homogeneity of the groups, using Cohen's d and phi coefficient (Φ) as measures of the effect sizes. 2 (Group) x 6 (Time) repeated measures analysis of variance (ANOVAs) were used to assess changes in clinical variables and psychosocial functioning, computing pairwise differences using Bonferroni correction. However, in those outcome variables in which the groups were not initially homogeneous, one-factor ANCOVAs were performed to analyze between-subjects differences controlling pretreatment levels. Partial eta-squared (η^2_p) was calculated to assess effect sizes for within and between-subjects' comparisons. All effect sizes were interpreted using the benchmarks provided by Cohen [36] (i.e., Cohen's d: small < 0.50, medium > 0.50 and < 0.80, and large > 0.80; Φ: small < 0.30, medium > 0.30 and < 0.50, and large > 0.50; η^2_p: small < 0.06, medium > 0.06 and < 0.14, and large > 0.14).

In addition, McNemar's tests were performed to determine the pre-post changes in the percentage of women with clinically significant scores and social variables in the two intervention formats.

3. Results

3.1. Adherence to Treatment

A total of 15 (28.30%) women dropped out of treatment, 13 during the sessions and 2 at follow-up. While the percentage of dropouts was higher in the group format than in the individual one (35.71% vs. 20%, respectively), this difference was not statistically significant ($\chi^2(1) = 0.92, p = 0.336, \Phi = 0.174$). Moreover, all the dropouts in the individual intervention occurred during the first four sessions, whereas two women in group intervention (7.14%) dropped-out at follow-up.

Regarding attendance at the sessions, significant differences were found ($\chi^2(1) = 6.12, p < 0.05$). As might be expected, all the women in the individual format attended all the sessions (since this was tailored to their availability), compared to 80% of attendance in the group intervention. There were no significant differences between groups in the performing homework, although it was higher for the individual intervention (95.90% vs. 89.24%).

Women's satisfaction with the program was high in both formats (individual M = 31; SD = 0.97; group M = 30.2; SD = 1.47), without significant differences between them in the total CSQ-8 score or in any of the eight assessed issues.

3.2. Sample Characteristics and Group Homogeneity

The mean age of the participants was 39.17 (SD = 10.19) years, ranging from 23 to 65. Most of them belonged to the middle social class (50.9%) and had completed primary (35.8%) or secondary studies (39.6%). 49.1% worked outside home, whereas 32.1% reported being housewives. More than one half of the samples (50.9%) were separated or underwent separation procedures, although about one third (30.2%) still lived with their aggressor at the time of the assessment, and 37.7% depended on him economically.

Regarding their history of maltreatment, it can be considered prolonged, with a mean of more than 11 years (M = 11.26; SD = 10.57), and of daily frequency in the past month for about 45% of the sample, with 45.3% classifying the current status of their problem as "the worst moment." Regarding the kind of maltreatment suffered, the most frequent (58.5%) was the combination of physical and psychological abuse; a great majority (96.23%) had suffered psychological abuse; physical abuse was also very common (66.04%); and sexual abuse was reported much less frequently (7.55%), and always in combination with psychological and/or physical abuse.

Sixty-four percent had presented charges about their situation, and about the half of the participants (52.8%) had to leave their home because of the violence. More than one third of the samples had received medical, psychological, or psychiatric attention because of the violence, and over 50% were taking medication (mainly antidepressant and anxiolytic drugs). In contrast, most of the women felt supported, principally by their families (79.2%), but also at a social (60.4%) and legal level (52.8%).

With regard to their emotional status, although none of the women met the diagnostic criteria for PTSD, as imposed by the inclusion criteria, 50.9% presented posttraumatic symptomatology above the EGS cut-off point, which indicates the clinical severity of these symptoms.

The women's mean depression score can be considered severe (according to the cut-off points established for the Spanish version of the scale), whereas the mean anxiety score was considered moderate–severe. Moreover, at the time of assessment, about half of the participants (50.9%) admitted having had suicide ideation. Likewise, the level of these women's self-esteem can be considered medium, and 50.9% of the interviewees were below this cut-off point. In contrast to these data, the mean alcohol consumption score was minimum, practically null for the total sample.

In order to assess groups homogeneity, group differences in sociodemographic variables, violence history, psychological health, and social issues were analyzed. As can be seen in Table 1, there were no statistically significant differences between the groups in sociodemographic variables and violence history. Regarding outcome variables, significant differences were observed in the mean levels of depression and anxiety, which were higher in the individual intervention. While the severity of the posttraumatic symptoms was also higher in the individual condition, differences did not reach statistical significance. In addition, participants in individual intervention also showed significantly lower scores in self-esteem. Finally, participants in the group format reported higher family and social support, although differences did not reach statistical significance.

Table 1. Characteristics of women, violence situation, emotional status, and groups homogeneity at baseline ($n = 53$).

	Individual ($n = 25$)	Group ($n = 28$)	Statistics	p	Effect Size
Age in years M (SD)	38.04 (10.53)	40.18 (9.95)	$t(51) = -0.76$	0.451	$d = 0.209$
Social class n (%)			Fisher exact test	0.071	-
Low	6 (24.0)	3 (10.7)			
Medium-low	4 (16.0)	9 (32.1)			
Medium	15 (60)	12 (42.9)			
Medium-high	0 (0.0)	4 (14.3)			
Marital status n (%)			Fisher exact test	0.454	-
Single	7 (28.0)	6 (21.4)			
Living with stable partner	3 (12.0)	1 (3.6)			
Married	2 (8.0)	6 (21.4)			
Divorced	13 (52.0)	14 (50.0)			
Widowed	0 (0.0)	1 (3.6)			
Work status n (%)			Fisher exact test	0.683	-
Active	5 (20.0)	8 (28.6)			
Unemployed	7 (28.0)	6 (21.4)			
Housewife	3 (12.0)	6 (21.4)			
Disabled	1 (4.0)	0 (0.0)			
Educational n (%)			Fisher exact test	0.269	-
Incomplete primary studies	5 (20.0)	1 (3.6)			
Complete primary studies	9 (36.0)	10 (35.7)			
Secondary level	9 (36.0)	12 (42.9)			
University level	2 (8.0)	5 (17.9)			
Lives with aggressor n (%)	7 (25.0)	9 (32.1)	$X^2(1,53) = 0.001$	0.977	$\Phi = 0.045$
Depends economically on aggressor n (%)	8 (32.0)	12 (42.9)	$X^2(1,53) = 0.28$	0.596	$\Phi = 0.112$
Duration (years) of maltreatment M (SD)	12.00 (10.89)	10.61 (10.42)	$t(51) = 0.48$	0.636	$d = 0.130$
Frequency of maltreatment past month n (%)			Fisher exact test	0.640	
Daily	9 (36.0)	15 (53.6)			
Once a week	3 (12.0)	2 (7.1)			
Once a month	5 (20.0)	5 (17.9)			
Has not occurred	8 (32.0)	6 (21.4)			
Type of maltreatment n (%)			Fisher exact test	0.080	-
Psychological	11 (44)	6 (21.4)			
Physical	0 (0.0)	1 (3.6)			
Psychological + Physical	12 (48)	19 (67.9)			
Psychological + Sexual	1 (4.0)	0 (0.0)			
Physical + Sexual	1 (4.0)	0 (0.0)			
Physical + Psychological + Sexual	0 (0.0)	2 (7.1)			
Has reported maltreatment n (%)	17 (68.0)	15 (53.6)	$X^2(1,53) = 0.62$	0.429	$\Phi = -0.147$
Has had to leave home n (%)	11 (44.0)	17 (60.7)	$X^2(1,53) = 0.89$	0.347	$\Phi = 0.167$
Medical attention n (%)	9 (36.9)	10 (35.7)	$X^2(1,53) = 0.00$	1.00	$\Phi = -0.003$
Psychiatric/psychological attention n (%)	7 (28.0)	13 (46.4)	$X^2(1,53) = 1.20$	0.272	$\Phi = 0.190$
Receives medication n (%)	13 (52.0)	15 (53.6)	$X^2(1,53) = 0.00$	1.00	$\Phi = 0.016$
Legal support n (%)	16 (64.0)	12 (42.9)	$X^2(1,53) = 1.60$	0.206	$\Phi = -0.211$
Family support n (%)	20 (80)	22 (78.6)	$X^2(1,53) = 0.00$	1.00	$\Phi = -0.018$
Social support n (%)	14 (56)	18 (63.3)	$X^2(1,53) = 0.11$	0.738	$\Phi = 0.085$
Suicidal ideation n (%)	10 (40.0)	17 (60.7)	$X^2(1,53) = 1.51$	0.218	$\Phi = 0.207$
Posttraumatic symptoms (EGS) M (SD) (0–51)	17.56 (6.44)	14.86 (6.51)	$t(51) = 1.51$	0.136	$d = 0.041$
Depression (BDI) M (SD) (0–63)	32.24 (12.61)	24.18 (14.03)	$t(51) = 2.08$	0.042	$d = 0.596$
Anxiety (BAI) M (SD) (0–63)	31.56 (11.83)	24.48 (12.54)	$t(51) = 2.05$	0.045	$d = 0.563$
Self-esteem (Rosenberg's) M (SD) (10–40)	25.80 (4,06)	28.00 (3.45)	$t(51) = -3.20$	0.002	$d = 0.874$
Alcohol consumption (CAGE) M (SD) (0–4)	0.08 (0.27)	0.14 (0.44)	$t(51) = -0.49$	0.042	$d = 0.136$

M = mean; SD = Standard Deviation; d = Cohen's d; Φ = phi coefficient; EGS = Severity of Posttraumatic Stress Disorder Symptoms Scale; BDI = Beck Depression Inventory; BAI = Beck Anxiety Inventory; Rosenberg's = Rosenberg's Self-Esteem Scale; CAGE = Cut-down, Annoyed, Guilty & Eye-opener.

3.3. Treatment Effectiveness

All the primary outcome variables and the secondary variable showed significant differences in time (Table 2). As can be seen in Figures 2–4, the means for posttraumatic symptoms, depression and anxiety show a pronounced and significant decrease between the baseline or pre-treatment values and the respective posttreatment values and these improvements are more or less sustained at the follow-ups ($p < 0.01$). In the case of self-esteem, the significant improvement ($p < 0.01$) delays until 1-month follow-up and is sustained from that moment (see Figure 5). All the effect sizes for time were large.

Table 2. Means, standard deviations and repeated measures ANOVA statistics for clinical variables ($n = 53$).

Variable	Individual ($n = 25$)		Group ($n = 28$)		ANOVA			
	M	SD	M	SD	Effect	F (1,51)	p	η^2_p
PTSD (EGS)								
Pretreatment	17.56	6.45	14.86	6.51	Group	0.30	0.584	0.006
Posttreatment	8.84	6.99	9.64	6.69	Time	65.15	<0.001	0.561
1 month	4.28	4.00	5.78	6.96	Group × Time	2.08	0.070	0.039
3 months	3.44	3.90	5.78	6.15				
6 months	4.04	3.72	4.86	5.83				
12 months	3.04	3.76	3.96	5.21				
Depression (BDI)								
Pretreatment	32.44	12.84	25.03	13.00	Group	0.06	0.801	0.001
Posttreatment	17.36	10.82	17.36	14.48	Time	41.58	<0.001	0.449
1 month	15.28	10.49	15.25	12.13	Group × Time	2.45	0.034	0.046
3 months	10.48	8.68	13.36	10.36				
6 months	9.48	7.30	10.39	10.37				
12 months	8.96	8.84	9.25	9.55				
Anxiety (BAI)								
Pretreatment	32.56	13.11	25.36	12.44	Group	0.079	0.780	0.002
Posttreatment	20.72	11.83	22.32	16.19	Time	35.13	<0.001	0.408
1 month	16.40	12.34	18.61	14.06	Group × Time	2.64	0.024	0.049
3 months	13.24	10.88	16.50	14.03				
6 months	10.76	9.21	12.14	8.43				
12 months	8.00	7.23	10.82	9.00				
Self-esteem (Rosenberg's)								
Pretreatment	25.12	4.05	28.28	3.12	Group	3.23	0.078	0.060
Posttreatment	28.68	3.21	28.64	4.18	Time	17.70	<0.001	0.258
1 month	29.40	3.01	31.50	3.40	Group × Time	1.52	0.184	0.029
3 months	30.68	3.14	31.64	5.00				
6 months	31.64	2.39	32.61	3.68				
12 months	30.28	5.47	30.93	6.02				

M = mean; SD = Standard Deviation; η^2_p = partial eta-square; EGS = Severity of Posttraumatic Stress Disorder Symptoms Scale; BDI = Beck Depression Inventory; BAI = Beck Anxiety Inventory; Rosenberg's = Rosenberg's Self-Esteem Scale.

More interestingly for the objectives of this study (Table 2), repeated measure ANOVAs did not reveal significant differences by group in the primary and secondary outcome variables. Given the differences observed between groups in pretreatment levels of depression, anxiety and self-esteem, we conducted one-factor ANCOVAs to control the possible effect of these differences in baseline measures. After controlling pretreatment values, no significant effects of group (depression: $F(1,50) = 0.620$, $p = 0.435$, $\eta^2_p = 0.012$; anxiety: $F(1,50) = 1.22$, $p = 0.274$, $\eta^2_p = 0.024$; self-esteem: $F(1,50) = 1.07$, $p = 0.307$, $\eta^2_p = 0.021$) or covariables (depression-pre: $F(1,50) = 2.69$ $p = 0.107$, $\eta^2_p = 0.051$; anxiety-pre: $F(1,50) = 1.22$, $p = 0.274$, $\eta^2_p = 0.024$; and self-esteem: $F(1,50) = 0.12$, $p = 0.912$, $\eta^2_p = 0.000$) emerged.

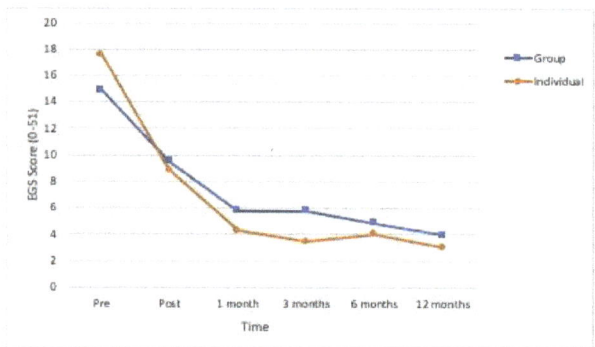

Figure 2. Evolution over time of the levels of posttraumatic symptoms (Severity of Posttraumatic Stress Disorder Symptoms Scale -EGS) in the two experimental conditions ($n = 53$).

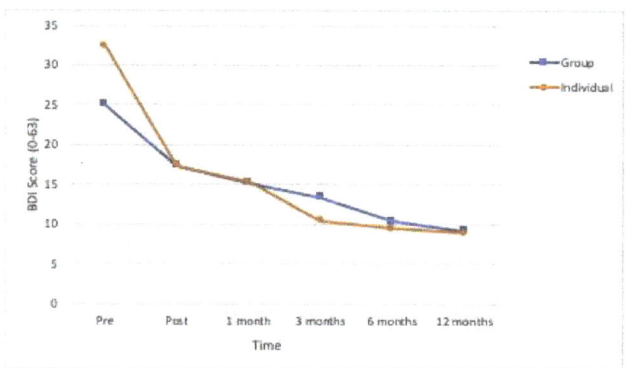

Figure 3. Evolution over time of the levels of depression (Beck Depression Inventory-BDI) in the two experimental conditions ($n = 53$).

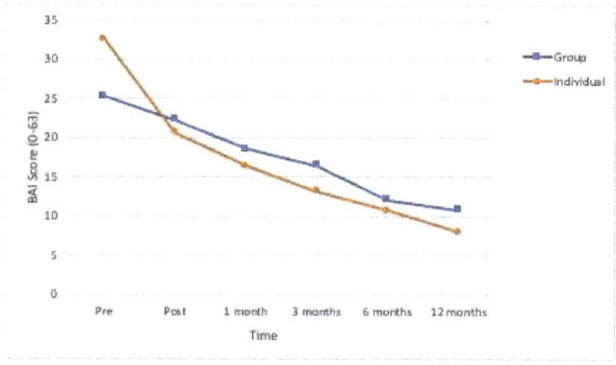

Figure 4. Evolution over time of the levels of anxiety (Beck Anxiety Inventory-BAI) in the two experimental conditions ($n = 53$).

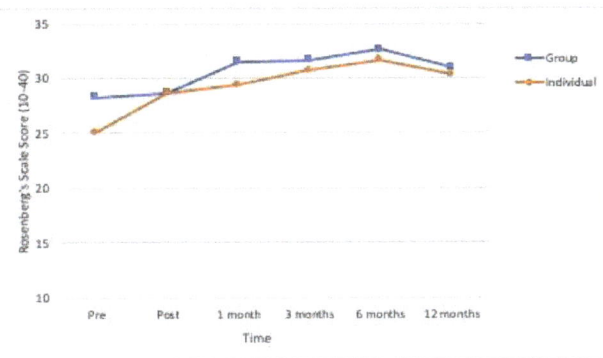

Figure 5. Evolution over time of the levels of self-esteem (Rosenberg's Self-Esteem Scale) in the two experimental conditions ($n = 53$).

We found a significant group x time interaction effect for depression and anxiety but not for posttraumatic symptoms and self-esteem (Table 2). Post-hoc comparisons revealed significant improvements in depressive symptoms from pretreatment to almost all the measures for both formats, although they showed a different pattern of improvement (Figure 3). The individual format showed a significant decrease in depressive symptoms between pretreatment and posttreatment ($p = 0.001$), which was maintained and then augmented at three-months follow-up, with significant differences between one and three-months follow-up ($p = 0.019$). In the group condition, there was also a significant decrease in depression symptoms from pretreatment to posttreatment ($p < 0.001$) and then from the six-months follow-up, with significant differences between posttreatment and 6- ($p = 0.002$) and 12-months ($p = -001$) follow-ups. Post-hoc comparisons did not reveal significant difference in depression between conditions in any of the times of measure.

Concerning anxiety (Figure 4), in the individual condition, we found a significant decrease in symptom severity from pre-treatment to post-treatment ($p = 0.010$), as well as to all follow-ups ($p < 0.001$ for all comparisons); symptoms showed a progressive decrease over time with significant differences between post-treatment to 6- ($p = 0.003$) and to 12-months follow-ups ($p < 0.001$), and between 1- and 12-months follow-ups ($p < 0.001$). The improvements in the group condition appeared to take much more time to emerge; although there was a progressive decrease in anxiety symptoms, it only reached statistical significance from the 6-months follow-up; specifically, the 6-months measure showed significant differences with posttreatment ($p < 0.001$) and 1-month follow-up ($p = 0.011$), while 12-months follow up showed significant differences with posttreatment ($p < 0.001$), 1- ($p < 0.001$) and 3-months follow-ups ($p = 0.019$). However, post-hoc comparisons did not reveal significant difference in anxiety between conditions in any of the times of measure.

From the clinical point of view, as observed in Table 3, there were important improvements in emotional status, with significant reduction in the percentages of women with possible problems of posttraumatic stress, depression, and anxiety in both intervention formats mainly in the long-term. While no significant differences were found between conditions in the percentage of women with clinically relevant posttraumatic, depressive and anxiety symptoms in the pre-treatment and each of the follow-up measures, individual treatment appears to have a slightly greater effect on symptoms. Specifically, McNemar's tests revealed that the individual condition promotes significant reduction in the rate of clinically meaningful PTSD symptoms from pretreatment to post-treatment ($p = 0.035$), 1-month ($p = 0.001$), 3-months ($p \leq 0.001$) and 12-months ($p < 0.001$) follow-ups. In the group condition significant improvements required more time. The proportion of women assigned to the group condition with clinically meaningful scores did not decline significantly from pre-treatment to post-treatment ($p = 0.424$) and from pre-treatment to 1-month follow-up ($p = 0.118$). However, there was a significant reduction of this proportion from pre-treatment to 3- ($p = 0.002$), 6- ($p = 0.003$) and 12-months ($p = 0.002$) follow-ups.

Table 3. Frequencies and comparisons between conditions in clinically significant symptomology and support ($n = 53$).

	Individual ($n = 25$)	Group ($n = 28$)	Statistics	p	Φ
Posttraumatic symptoms (EGS) n (%)					
Pretreatment	15 (60)	12 (42.9)	$X^2 (1,53) = 0.94$	0.332	−0.171
Posttreatment	6 (24.0)	8 (28.6)	$X^2 (1,53) = 0.004$	0.948	0.052
1 month	1 (4.0)	5 (17.9)	Fisher exact test	0.196	-
3 months	1 (4.0)	2 (7.1)	Fisher exact test	1.00	-
6 months	0 (0.0)	1 (3.6)	Fisher exact test	1.00	-
12 months	1 (4.0)	2 (7.1)	Fisher exact test	1.00	-
Depression (BDI) n (%)					
Pretreatment	24 (96.0)	23 (82.1)	$X^2 (1,53) = 1.33$	0.248	−0.218
Posttreatment	15 (60.0)	13 (46.4)	$X^2 (1,53) = 0.51$	0.476	−0.136
1 month	11 (44.0)	10 (35.7)	$X^2 (1,53) = 0.11$	0.738	−0.085
3 months	7 (28.0)	11 (29.3)	$X^2 (1,53) = 0.33$	0.565	0.119
6 months	7 (28.0)	8 (28.6)	$X^2 (1,53) = 0.00$	1.00	0.006
12 months	5 (20.0)	6 (21.4)	$X^2 (1,53) = 0.00$	1.00	0.018
Anxiety (BAI) n (%)					
Pretreatment	24 (96.0)	21 (75.0)	$X^2 (1,53) = 3.05$	0.081	−0.293
Posttreatment	19 (76.0)	17 (60.7)	$X^2 (1,53) = 0.80$	0.371	−0.163
1 month	15 (60.0)	16 (57.1)	$X^2 (1,53) = 0.00$	1.00	−0.029
3 months	9 (36.0)	14 (50.0)	$X^2 (1,53) = 0.56$	0.454	0.141
6 months	10 (40.0)	12 (42.9)	$X^2 (1,53) = 0.00$	1.00	0.029
12 months	7 (28.0)	12 (42.9)	$X^2 (1,53) = 0.70$	0.401	0.155
Family support n (%)					
Pretreatment	20 (80.0)	22 (78.6)	$X^2 (1,53) = 0.00$	1.00	−0.018
Posttreatment	18 (72.0)	22 (78.6)	$X^2 (1,53) = 0.05$	0.814	0.076
1 month	18 (72.0)	25 (89.3)	$X^2 (1,53) = 1.57$	0.210	0.221
3 months	21 (84.0)	20 (71.4)	$X^2 (1,53) = 0.58$	0.446	−0.150
6 months	18 (72.0)	22 (78.6)	$X^2 (1,53) = 0.05$	0.814	0.076
12 months	17 (68.0)	18 (64.3)	$X^2 (1,53) = 0.00$	1.00	−0.039
Social support n (%)					
Pretreatment	14 (56.9)	18 (64.3)	$X^2 (1,53) = 0.11$	0.738	0.085
Posttreatment	22 (88.0)	24 (85.7)	$X^2 (1,53) = 0.00$	1.00	−0.034
1 month	19 (76.0)	23 (82.1)	$X^2 (1,53) = 0.04$	0.833	0.076
3 months	21 (84.0)	18 (64.3)	$X^2 (1,53) = 1.72$	0.189	−0.223
6 months	20 (80.0)	19 (67.9)	$X^2 (1,53) = 0.47$	0.491	−0.137
12 months	22 (88.0)	23 (82.1)	$X^2 (1,53) = 0.04$	0.833	−0.082

Φ = phi coefficient; EGS = Severity of Posttraumatic Stress Disorder Symptoms Scale; BDI = Beck Depression Inventory; BAI = Beck Anxiety Inventory.

Regarding depression, both conditions promote significant decline in the proportion of participants with clinical meaningful scores from pre-treatment to post-treatment (individual: $p = 0.012$; group: $p = 0.006$), 1-month (individual: $p = 0.001$; group: $p = 0.001$), 3-months (individual: $p \leq 0.001$; group: $p = 0.002$), 6-months (individual: $p \leq 0.001$; group: $p < 0.001$) and 12-months (individual: $p \leq 0.001$; group: $p < 0.001$) follow-ups.

Finally, although individual intervention promotes a significant reduction in clinically meaningful anxious symptomatology from pre-treatment to all other measures (post-treatment: $p = 0.012$; 1-mont: $p = 0.012$; 3-months: $p \leq 0.001$; 6-months: $p = 0.001$; 12-months: $p < 0.001$), group condition only showed a significant decline of this proportion from pre-treatment to post-treatment ($p = 0.006$), 6-months ($p = 0.022$) and 12-months ($p = 0.022$) measures.

3.4. Effect of Individual and Group Formats on Social Variables

Finally, to test the effect of both formats of treatment on social issues, the progression in the perception of familiar and social support was analyzed. It is worth mentioning that, in pre-treatment assessment, most women in both conditions showed family support, and to a lesser extent, also social support (Table 1)

Regarding treatment effects, no significant variations were found between pre-treatment and follow-ups in the presence or absence of family support in both the individual and in the group condition. Moreover, as can be seen in Table 3, no significant differences between conditions were found at any time measure.

Conversely, treatment promoted significant improvements on perceived social support. In the individual condition, there were significant differences from pretreatment to posttreatment ($p = 0.008$), 3-months ($p = 0.039$) and 12-months follow-ups ($p = 0.039$). Specifically, among women that did not reported social support at pretreatment, 72.7% had it at posttreatment and 3-months follow-up and 90.9% at 12-months follow-up. In the group condition, the variations in social support only approached significance at a short-term ($p = 0.007$), given the 70% of participants that did not report social support at pretreatment and did it at posttreatment. Otherwise, no significant differences were found when comparing pretreatment reports and all other measures (1-month: $p = 0.180$; 3-months: $p = 1.00$; 6-months: $p = 1.00$: 12-months: $p = 0.302$). Nevertheless, as can be seen in Table 3, no significant differences between conditions were found at any time measure.

4. Discussion

This study compares individual vs. group formats of a CBT trauma-focused intervention that has previously shown its effectiveness for women victims of IPV with sub-clinical PTSD symptoms [16]. Further, it specifically analyses the effect of both formats on social issues, which has been claimed to be an advantage for group interventions [13,14]. In this way, it provides valuable information for the design of resources and the implementation of interventions to improve emotional state and psychopathological symptoms in female survivors of IPV.

The data show that the trauma-focused CBT proposed herein (both intervention formats) has a significant effect, with significant reductions in posttraumatic, depression and anxiety symptoms in women that have suffered severe and long-lasting IPV (over 10 years in both groups); for all these variables, the changes emerge at posttreatment and are maintained in the follow-ups up to one year after intervention. In addition, it also achieved significant improvement in self-esteem that becomes significant since 1-month follow-up. Moreover, data show a significant clinical effect with significant decreases in the percentages of women with clinically significant emotional problems [37].

According to Arroyo et al. [10] findings, the effect of both interventions was higher in posttraumatic symptomatology. However, this result contrasts with the recent Cochrane Review by Hameed et al. [38], where, according to the computed effect sizes, it was concluded that, although psychological therapies probably reduce depression and may reduce anxiety symptoms in IPV survivors at medium-term (6 to 12 months), there is no certainty about their beneficial effect on PTSD symptoms. While our findings also point to larger effect sizes in the reduction of depression and anxiety symptoms intensity, the discrepancy with the Cochrane Review [38] regarding PTSD symptomatology may respond to certain methodological differences. First of all, although our treatment combined different techniques, it constituted a trauma-focused intervention and the larger effect on PTSD symptoms is coherent with its main objective. By contrast, the above-mentioned reviews include different types of interventions on the basis of more flexible or broad inclusion and exclusion criteria. While Hameed et al. [38] started their review from a clear clinical definition of the psychotherapy concept, Arroyo et al. [10] considered a wider definition, including some less clinical and structured techniques like yogic breathing or counseling. Moreover, participants in our study and across all studies reviewed by Arroyo et al. [10] were heterosexual females abused by men, whereas Hameed et al. [37] included some studies with a minor proportion of women who report IPV perpetrated by a same-sex partner. In addition, contrary to the face-to-face and brief nature of our intervention and all treatments included by Arroyo et al. [10], Hameed et al. [38] did not establish these restrictions. Nevertheless, our study responds precisely to the need claimed in these reviews of further research with consistent methodologies to increase the evidence-based knowledge about the intervention with IPV survivors.

The treatment accomplished long-term effects, enabling women to handle trauma derived from IPV; moreover, improvements consolidated and even increased over time. These results are in line with those obtained with different versions of this trauma-focused CBT in group format (e.g., [16,20,39–41]) and with other CBT in individual format [42] or individual and combined one (i.e., individual + group; Echeburúa et al. [11]), and point that trauma-focused CBT can meet the demands and needs of female survivors of IPV, improving, clinically and significantly, their emotional status.

The good effect of treatment could be limited by the high percentage of dropouts (28.3%), which, however, is similar to that of other interventions (e.g., Kubany et al. [42]: 20% in individual format). As well as the lack of motivation, these high rates may be related to the specific circumstances of these women (i.e., undergoing a transition period with frequent changes of home, work status, etc.). Moreover, the higher percentage of dropouts in the group format (37.71% vs. 20% in individual) may relate to the difficulties for flexibility in the schedule and access to the sessions. Nonetheless, neither this difference, neither differences between formats in the accomplishment of homework nor satisfaction with therapy reached statistical significance, which would support the implementation of the group format.

In this line, and against initial predictions and previous results (cf. Arroyo et al. [10]), there were only marginal significant differences between both delivery formats. While Fernández-Velasco [12], applying this same program to women with PTSD diagnosis, reported that the individual format was superior to group intervention, mainly at 6- and 12-months follow-ups, in this study both formats obtained similar effects, and differences tended to decrease over time, until almost disappearing at 6-months and mostly 12-months follow-ups. Discrepancies between present results and Fernández-Velasco's [12], who focused on women with PTSD diagnosis, could point that individual format poses some advantages for IPV survivors with a more severe emotional impact (namely, PTSD diagnosis). It should be noted that Echeburúa et al. [11], when comparing individual vs. individual + group formats, found that combined therapy did better than the individual one in PTSD symptoms and impaired functioning at follow-up assessment, partially supporting the beneficial effects of group therapy as adjunctive to individual CBT.

Furthermore, contrary to expectations, the group format did not present any advantage to get family or social support. In fact, neither of the two formats appear to have any effect on family support. Conversely, although no differences were found between formats in social support, the individual treatment promotes significant short- and long-term improvements, whereas, in the group condition, the variations in social support only approached significance in the short-term. Maybe a close therapeutic bond established in the individual treatment might be more powerful than social encouragement provided by the group, which could have a limited effect that disappears once the therapy is finished. In addition, it should be taken into account that women in the present study had a good initial level of social and family support, which could have provoked a "ceiling effect"; the analysis of this element in highly isolated women is thus open to further research.

The study complies with most of the requirements for research on treatments outcomes [19]: a well-trained psychologist delivered the interventions, using manualized protocols, which would facilitate their future application; random assignment of participants to the experimental conditions; in-depth assessment; a fixed number of sessions; and inclusion of long-term follow-up. Nonetheless, some limitations of the study must be pointed out. First, the generalization of results is potentially limited by the fact that all treatments were applied by the same therapist; even though the use of a manualized protocol could contribute to mitigate potential biases. Secondly, the evaluations were not performed by blind interviews. Thirdly, the small sample size, mainly at the follow-ups, could have implications for statistical power. Finally, the study does not include a control group; although a waiting-list control group was initially planned, it was finally discarded since, in the pilot study, none of the women from the waiting-list subsequently entered treatment [34], and due to the ethical considerations of giving women no access to the intervention that they demand and may be a crucial tool for their recovery. Nonetheless, the inclusion of a comparison group with treatment as usual should be considered for the future. Likewise, the inclusion of women who still live with their abuser could be questioned.

All in all, this study has significant clinical implications. It provides additional support of a brief trauma-focused therapy (eight session) that have proved to be effective in the reduction of symptoms and discomfort in IPV survivors with significant posttraumatic symptoms; actually, it has been included as such in several recent reviews on this topic (cf. [10,43–45]). Furthermore, since data do not show significant differences between individual and group delivery formats, or in symptoms reduction or in dropouts, group application of this treatment emerges as a therapeutic alternative that could be very helpful due to its cost-effectiveness advantage over individual modalities.

Future research should focus on the adequacy of the format to symptoms severity as well as on the consideration of other variables (e.g., cohabitation with the abuser, availability of social support, motivation for the change, etc.) that would affect the effect of the format; some of them, though included in this study, has not been analyzed due to the small sample size that would affect statistical power and prevent methodologically safe conclusions. Similarly, effect of group format should be tested in IPV survivors that lack social support, since the beneficial social effect of group interaction promoted by this format could arise and gain relevance in isolated women. Moreover, the inclusion of the combined format (i.e., including some individual and some group sessions) could offer a promising path that would deserve attention, considering the individual and group formats not only as alternatives but also as complements.

5. Conclusions

Cognitive-behavioral trauma focused intervention for IPV survivor delivered in the group format proved effective in symptom reduction as an individual format, with no significant increase in dropouts. While it did not seem to imply any advantage in social issues, since it would maintain a good cost-effectiveness balance, it would be a relevant alternative for community, social and clinical services, frequently overloaded, allowing for considerable savings in cost, time and efforts. Nevertheless, the careful analysis of each woman needs and circumstances (e.g., schedule availability, motivation for change, difficulties to sharing emotions and problems, isolation or availability of social support, severity of symptoms, etc.) must prevail as a guide for the choice of the delivery format.

Author Contributions: Conceptualization, M.C. and M.A.; Methodology, M.C., M.A. and C.S.; Formal Analysis, M.C., M.A. and C.S.; Investigation, M.C. and M.A.; Resources, M.C.; Data Curation, M.C., M.A. and C.S.; Writing—Original Draft Preparation, M.C., M.A. and C.S.; Writing—Review & Editing, M.C.; Visualization, C.S.; Supervision, M.C.; Project Administration, M.C.; Funding Acquisition, M.C., M.A. and C.S. All authors have read and agreed to the published version of the manuscript.

Funding: This research was supported by the Spanish Ministry of Economy and Competitiveness (PSI2012-31952), by the Santander-Complutense University Project PR75/18-21569, and by the Spanish Ministry of Science and Innovation (PID2019-105942RB-I00), and by scholarships from the Spanish Ministry of Education to M. Arinero and from the Universidad Complutense de Madrid to C. Soberón.

Institutional Review Board Statement: The study was conducted according to the guidelines of the Declaration of Helsinki, and approved by the Ethics Committee of Psychology Faculty, Universidad Complutense de Madrid (number 2016/17-022).

Informed Consent Statement: Informed consent was obtained from all subjects involved in this study.

Data Availability Statement: The data presented in this study are available on request from the corresponding author.

Acknowledgments: We would like to thank Francisco J. Labrador and Paulina P. Rincón for their collaboration in the development of the project, for the access to the participants, and for performing numerous assessments of the potential participants. We also thank to all the women involved in this study as well as the institutions that recruited participants and facilitated the development of the program in their centers: The Council for Women and Elderly of the City Council of Collado-Villalba, the Women's Services of the City Council of Toledo, The Victims' Assistance Offices of Móstoles and Coslada, the Rosa of Luxembourg Women's Center of Leganés, and The Social Services Center of Entrevías.

Conflicts of Interest: The authors declare no conflict of interests.

References

1. World Health Organization; Department of Reproductive Health and Research; London School of Hygiene and Tropical Medicine; South African Medical Research Council. *Global and Regional Estimates of Violence against Women: Prevalence and Health Effects of Intimate Partner Violence and Non-Partner Sexual Violence*; World Health Organization: Geneva, Switzerland, 2013.
2. Domenech, I.; Sirvent, E. The consequences of intimate partner violence on health: A further disaggregation of psychological violence-evidence from Spain. *Violence Women* **2017**, *23*, 1771–1789. [CrossRef]
3. Smith, S.G.; Zhang, X.; Basile, K.C.; Merrick, M.T.; Wang, J.; Kresnow, M.; Chen, J. *The National Intimate Partner and Sexual Violence Survey (NISVS): 2015 Data Brief—Updated Release*; National Center for Injury Prevention, and Control, Centers for Disease Control and Prevention: Atlanta, GA, USA, 2018.
4. Lagdon, S.; Armour, C.; Stringer, M. Adult experience of mental health outcomes as a result of intimate partner violence victimisation: A systematic review. *Eur. J. Psychotraumatol.* **2014**, *5*, 24794. [CrossRef]
5. Koenen, K.C.; Ratanatharathorn, A.; Ng, L.; McLaughlin, K.A.; Bromet, E.J.; Stein, D.J.; Karam, E.G.; Ruscio, A.M.; Benjet, C.; Scott, K.; et al. Posttraumatic stress disorder in the world mental health surveys. *Psychol. Med.* **2017**, *47*, 2260–2274. [CrossRef]
6. Coker, A.L.; Davis, K.E.; Arias, I.; Desai, S.; Sanderson, M.; Brandt, H.M.; Smith, P.H. Physical and mental health effects of intimate partner violence for men and women. *Am. J. Prev. Med.* **2002**, *23*, 260–268. [CrossRef]
7. Pico-Alfonso, M.A.; Garcia-Linares, M.I.; Celda-Navarro, N.; Blasco-Ros, C.; Echeburúa, E.; Martinez, M. The impact of physical, psychological, and sexual intimate male partner violence on women's mental health: Depressive symptoms, posttraumatic stress disorder, state anxiety, and suicide. *J. Women's Health* **2006**, *15*, 599–611. [CrossRef]
8. Nathanson, A.M.; Shorey, R.C.; Tirone, V.; Rhatigan, D.L. The prevalence of mental health disorders in a community sample of female victims of intimate partner violence. *Partn. Abus.* **2012**, *3*, 59–75. [CrossRef] [PubMed]
9. Helfrich, C.A.; Fujiura, G.T.; Rutkowski-Kmitta, V. Mental health disorders and functioning of women in domestic violence shelters. *J. Interpers. Violence* **2008**, *23*, 437–453. [CrossRef]
10. Arroyo, K.; Lundahl, B.; Butters, R.; Vanderloo, M.; Wood, D.S. Short-term interventions for survivors of intimate partner violence: A systematic review and meta-analysis. *Trauma Violence Abus.* **2017**, *18*, 155–171. [CrossRef] [PubMed]
11. Echeburúa, E.; Sarasua, B.; Zubizarreta, I. Individual versus individual and group therapy regarding a cognitive-behavioral treatment for battered women in a community setting. *J. Interpers. Violence* **2014**, *29*, 1783–1801. [CrossRef]
12. Fernández-Velasco, M.R. Estrés Postraumático y Violencia de Pareja: Análisis de la Eficacia de Tratamientos Psicológicos. Ph.D. Dissertation, Universidad Complutense de Madrid, Madrid, Spain, 2014.
13. Miller, L.E.; Howell, K.H.; Graham-Bermann, S.A. The effect of an evidence-based intervention on women's exposure to intimate partner violence. *Am. J. Orthopsychiatry* **2014**, *84*, 321–328. [CrossRef] [PubMed]
14. Graham-Bermann, S.A.; Miller, L.E. Intervention to reduce traumatic stress following intimate partner violence: An efficacy trial of the moms' empowerment program (MEP). *Psychodyn. Psychiatry* **2013**, *41*, 329–349. [CrossRef] [PubMed]
15. Foy, D.W.; Glynn, S.M.; Schnurr, P.P.; Jankowski, M.K.; Wattenberg, M.S.; Weiss, D.S.; Gusman, F.D. Group therapy. In *Effective Treatments for PTSD: Practice Guidelines from the International Society for Traumatic Stress Studies*; Foa, E.B., Keane, T.M., Friedman, M.J., Eds.; Guilford Press: New York, NY, USA, 2000; pp. 336–338.
16. Crespo, M.; Arinero, M. Assessment of the efficacy of a psychological treatment for women victims of violence by their intimate male partner. *Span. J. Psychol.* **2010**, *13*, 849–863. [CrossRef]
17. Echeburúa, E.; De Corral, P.; Amor, P.J.; Zubizarreta, I.; Sarasua, B. Escala de gravedad de síntomas del trastorno de estrés postraumático: Propiedades psicométricas [Posttraumatic stress symptom severity scale: Psychometric properties]. *Anál. Modif. Conducta* **1997**, *23*, 503–526.

18. American Psychiatric Association. *Diagnostic and Statistical Manual of Mental Disorders: DSM-IV-TR*; American Psychiatric Association: Washington, DC, USA, 2000.
19. Schulz, K.F.; Altman, D.G.; Moher, D. CONSORT 2010 statement: Updated guidelines for reporting parallel group randomised trials. *BMJ* **2010**, *340*, C332. [CrossRef]
20. Rincón, P.P.; Labrador, F.J. Transtorno de estrés postraumático en víctimas de maltrato doméstico: Evaluación de un programa de intervención [Posttraumatic stress disorder in victims of domestic violence: Assessment of an intervention program]. *Anál. Modif. Conducta* **2002**, *28*, 905–934.
21. Ewing, J.A. Detecting alcoholism. The CAGE questionnaire. *JAMA* **1984**, *252*, 1905–1907. [CrossRef]
22. Fonseca del Pozo, F.J.; Pérula de Torres, L.Á.; Martínez de La Iglesia, J. Detección de alcoholismo en una población general a través de la aplicación del test de Cage [The detection of alcoholism in a general population by using the CAGE test]. *Aten. Primaria* **1993**, *11*, 393–399.
23. Rodríguez-Martos, A.; Navarro, R.; Vecino, C.; Pérez, R. Validación de los cuestionarios KFA (CBA) y CAGE para el diagnóstico del alcoholismo [Validation of KFA (CBA) and CAGE in the diagnosis of alcoholism]. *Drogalcohol* **1986**, *11*, 132–139.
24. Beck, A.T.; Steer, R.A.; Brown, G.K. *BDI–II. Beck Depression Inventory–Second Edition Manual*; The Psychological Corporation: San Antonio, TX, USA, 1996.
25. Sanz, J.; Navarro, M.E.; Vázquez, C. Adaptación española del Inventario para la Depresión de Beck—II (BDI-II): 1. Propiedades psicométricas en estudiantes universitarios [Spanish adaptation of the Beck Depression Inventory-II (BDI-II): 1. Psychometric properties with university students]. *Anál. Notif. Conducta* **2003**, *29*, 239–288.
26. Sanz, J.; Perdigón, A.L.; Vázquez, C. Adaptación española del Inventario para la Depresión de Beck-II (BDI-II): 2. Propiedades psicométricas en población general [The Spanish adaptation of Beck´s Depression Inventory-II (BDI-II): 2. Psychometric properties in the general population]. *Clín. Salud.* **2003**, *14*, 249–280.
27. Sanz, J.; García-Vera, M.P.; Espinosa, R.; Fortún, M.; Vázquez, C. Adaptación española del Inventario para la Depresión de Beck-II (BDI-II): 3. Propiedades psicométricas en pacientes con trastornos psicológicos [Spanish adaptation of the Beck Depression Inventory-II (BDI-II): 3. Psychometric features in patients with psychological disorders]. *Clín. Salud.* **2005**, *16*, 121–142.
28. Beck, A.T.; Epstein, N.; Brown, G.; Steer, R.A. An inventory for measuring clinical anxiety: Psychometric properties. *J. Consult. Clin. Psychol.* **1988**, *56*, 893–897. [CrossRef] [PubMed]
29. Sanz, J.; Navarro, M.E. Propiedades psicométricas de una versión española del inventario de ansiedad de beck (BAI) en estudiantes universitarios [The psychometric properties of a spanish version of the Beck Anxiety Inventory (BAI) in a university students' sample]. *Ansiedad Estrés* **2003**, *9*, 59–84.
30. Sanz, J. Recomendaciones para la utilización de la adaptación española del Inventario de Ansiedad de Beck (BAI) en la práctica clínica [Recommendations for the use of the Spanish adaptation of the Beck Anxiety Inventory (BAI) in clinical practice]. *Clín. Salud.* **2014**, *25*, 39–48. [CrossRef]
31. Rosenberg, A. *Society and the Adolescent Self-Image*; Princeton University Press: Princeton, NJ, USA, 1965.
32. Echeburúa, E.; Corral, P. *Manual de Violencia Familiar [Family Violence Handbook]*; Pirámide: Madrid, Spain, 1998.
33. Larsen, D.L.; Attkisson, C.C.; Hargreaves, W.A.; Nguyen, T.D. Assessment of client/patient satisfaction: Development of a general scale. *Eval. Program Plan.* **1979**, *2*, 197–207. [CrossRef]
34. Arinero, M.; Crespo, M. Evaluación de la eficacia de un programa de tratamiento psicológico para mujeres víctimas de maltrato doméstico: Estudio piloto [Assessment of the efficacy of a psychological program for female victims of domestic violence: Pilot study]. *Psicol. Conduct.* **2004**, *12*, 233–249.
35. Little, R.J.A. A test of missing completely at random for multivariate data with missing values. *J. Am. Stat. Assoc.* **1988**, *83*, 1198–1202. [CrossRef]
36. Cohen, J. *Statistical Power Analysis for the Behavioral Sciences*; Lawrence Earlbaum Associates: Hillsdale, NJ, USA, 1988.
37. Jacobson, N.S.; Roberts, L.J.; Berns, S.B.; McGlinchey, J.B. Methods for defining and determining the clinical significance of treatment effects: Description, application, and alternatives. *J. Consult. Clin. Psychol.* **1999**, *67*, 300–307. [CrossRef] [PubMed]
38. Hameed, M.; O'Doherty, L.; Gilchrist, G.; Tirado-Muñoz, J.; Taft, A.; Chondros, P.; Feder, G.; Tan, M.; Hegarty, K. Psychological therapies for women who experience intimate partner violence. *Cochrane Database Syst. Rev.* **2020**, *7*, CD013017. [CrossRef]
39. Alonso, E.; Labrador, F.J. Eficacia de un programa de intervención para el trastorno de estrés postraumático en mujeres inmigrantes víctimas de violencia de pareja: Un estudio piloto [Effectiveness of a treatment program for immigrant women victims of partner violence, with postraumatic stress disorder: A pilot estudy]. *Interam. J. Psychol.* **2010**, *44*, 547–559.
40. Cáceres, E. Tratamiento Psicológico Centrado en el Trauma en Mujeres Víctimas de Violencia de Pareja. Ph.D. Dissertation, Universidad Complutense de Madrid, Madrid, Spain, 2012.
41. Labrador, F.J.; Alonso, E. Eficacia a corto plazo de un programa de intervención para el trastorno de estrés postraumático en mujeres mexicanas víctimas de violencia doméstica [Short term effectiveness of a treatment program for the posttraumatic stress disorder in Mexican women victims of domestic violence]. *Rev. Psicopat. Psicol. Clín.* **2007**, *12*, 117–130. [CrossRef]
42. Kubany, E.S.; Hill, E.E.; Owens, J.A. Cognitive trauma therapy for battered women with PTSD: Preliminary findings. *J. Trauma Stress* **2003**, *16*, 81–91. [CrossRef] [PubMed]
43. Menon, B.; Stoklosa, H.; Van Dommelen, K.; Awerbuch, A.; Caddell, L.; Roberts, K.; Potter, J. Informing human trafficking clinical care through two systematic reviews on sexual assault and intimate partner violence. *Trauma Violence Abus.* **2020**, *21*, 932–945. [CrossRef] [PubMed]

44. Trabold, N.; McMahon, J.; Alsobrooks, S.; Whitney, S.; Mittal, M. A systematic review of intimate partner violence interventions: State of the field and implications for practitioners. *Trauma Violence Abus.* **2020**, *21*, 311–325. [CrossRef] [PubMed]
45. Warshaw, C.; Sullivan, C.M. *A Systematic Review of Trauma-Focused Interventions for Domestic Violence Survivors*; National Center on Domestic Violence, Trauma & Mental Health: East Lansing, MI, USA, 2013.

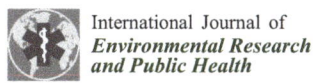

Article

Responses to Stress: Investigating the Role of Gender, Social Relationships, and Touch Avoidance in Italy

Marcello Passarelli [1,*], Laura Casetta [2], Luca Rizzi [2] and Raffaella Perrella [3]

[1] Institute of Educational Technology, National Research Council of Italy, 16149 Genova, Italy
[2] Associazione Centro di Psicologia e Psicoterapia Funzionale, 35131 Padova, Italy; l.casetta@psicoterapiafunzionale.it (L.C.); l.rizzi@psicoterapiafunzionale.it (L.R.)
[3] Department of Psychology, University of Campania "Luigi Vanvitelli", 81100 Caserta, Italy; raffaella.perrella@unicampania.it
* Correspondence: passarelli@itd.cnr.it

Abstract: Stress is a physiological response to internal and external events we call "stressors". Response to the same daily stressors varies across individuals and seems to be higher for women. A possible explanation for this phenomenon is that women perceive sociality, relationships, and intimacy—important sources of both stress and wellbeing—differently from how men experience them. In this study, we investigate how gender, attachment, and touch avoidance predict stress responses on a sample of 335 Italians (216 females; age = 35.82 ± 14.32). Moreover, we analyze the network of relationships between these variables through multiple linear regression and exploratory network analysis techniques. The results recontextualize the role of gender in determining stress responses in terms of (lack of) confidence and touch avoidance toward family members; attitudes toward relationships seem to be the main determinants of stress responses. These results have implications for reducing stress in both clinical settings and at a social level.

Keywords: stress response; gender differences; social behavior; attachment; touch avoidance; network analysis

Citation: Passarelli, M.; Casetta, L.; Rizzi, L.; Perrella, R. Responses to Stress: Investigating the Role of Gender, Social Relationships, and Touch Avoidance in Italy. *Int. J. Environ. Res. Public Health* **2021**, *18*, 600. https://doi.org/10.3390/ijerph18020600

Received: 4 November 2020
Accepted: 10 January 2021
Published: 12 January 2021

Publisher's Note: MDPI stays neutral with regard to jurisdictional claims in published maps and institutional affiliations.

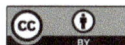

Copyright: © 2021 by the authors. Licensee MDPI, Basel, Switzerland. This article is an open access article distributed under the terms and conditions of the Creative Commons Attribution (CC BY) license (https://creativecommons.org/licenses/by/4.0/).

1. Introduction

Selye was the first to use the term stress to refer to a "response" elicited by a stimulus called a stressor [1,2]. As defined by Everly and Lating, "stress is a physiological response that serves as a mechanism of mediation linking any given stressor to its target-organ effect." [3–5].

Stressor events can be psychosocial and biogenic [3]. Psychosocial stressors are either real or imagined environmental events that lay the ground for the elicitation of the stress response. Biogenic stressors, instead, actually "cause" the elicitation of the stress response. Examples of such stimuli include caffeine, amphetamines, and guarana.

Individuals respond differently to the same stressors due to both biological and psychological individual characteristics [6]. In clinical practice, therapists usually intervene in how psychosocial stressors are perceived and managed.

Analyzing previous studies on influences on stress, it has been found that gender is an important variable in predicting stress responses. Specifically, several studies have highlighted that women, on average, report higher chronic stress and somatic symptoms than men, even when exposed to the same stressors [7,8]. This result has led to diverging interpretations, speculating on the reasons behind this gender difference. One such interpretation of gender differences in stress responses may be found in how males and females behave in social contexts, displaying different behaviors as well as different attitudes regarding social relationships, social touch, and intimacy.

Since social relationships are a source of both stress and wellbeing, and attachment and intimacy are keystones for mental health for both men and women [9,10], the intention of this study is to provide clinicians with a better understanding of the mechanisms behind the stress-response process so as to improve effective treatments of stress-related disorders and to reduce their cost and length. In particular, in this study, we will investigate the following research questions in the Italian population:

RQ1—Do gender, attachment dimensions, and attitudes towards touch predict the self-reported intensity of stress responses?

RQ2—How are gender, attachment dimensions, attitudes towards touch, and stress-responses interrelated?

While RQ1 is a more traditional approach to finding predictors, the exploratory nature of RQ2 has the aim of shedding light on the complex web of relationships between these variables. There is considerable evidence that gender, attachment, attitudes towards touch, and stress responses are interrelated, but the literature is fragmented and studies often consider a single pair of variables. In this study, we will try to gain a bird's eye view of how individual characteristics interact and influence stress responses, with the aim of guiding the planning of psychological interventions.

In the following sections, we will discuss the rationale for considering gender, attachment, and attitudes towards touch as important predictors of stress.

1.1. Examining Gender Differences in Social Behaviors from an Evolutionary Perspective

According to the biosocial model by Wood and Eagly [11], gender differences in social behavior are driven by two factors: physical differences and sociocultural influences.

Physical differences include women's ability to bear and nurse children and men's greater strength, speed, and size, which lead to women lending more parental care than men. Paternity uncertainty and mating opportunity cost hypotheses further explain gender differences in providing paternal care [12]. The former implies that since fathers are never certain that the offspring they are raising are genetically related to them, they perceive higher cost and risk in investing in parental care. The mating opportunity cost hypothesis, additionally, highlights that males that provide extensive parental care incur an opportunity cost since they could invest those resources in mating with a variety of females, thus having more children and spreading their genetic code further [12].

Studies on gender differences in social behavior seem to confirm that men, on average, invest less in their relationships (including nonpaternal relationships). According to an extensive literature review [13], men generally emphasize instrumentality and independence, whereas women value inclusiveness and interdependence. Indeed, males spend more money to elevate their status and favor promotions that benefit their status, suggesting they are more self-oriented as a short-term sexual strategy [12,13]. In contrast, women favor resources that benefit both themselves and others and are more aware of how their actions affect others; they are also more inclined to help others and to use social support to cope with negative emotions [7,14]. These findings suggest that, overall, women are more other-oriented than men [13].

We could, therefore, hypothesize that gender differences in stress originate from what women value most: caring for others. Indeed, minor daily stressors seem to impact women more than men, and the former more often report family- and health-related events that are experienced by other people as being stressful in their environment. On the other hand, men report out-of-family relationships, work, and finances as having a negative impact on their wellbeing [7].

1.2. How Relationship Bonds Are Created and Maintained: The Role of Touch

Even if social behavior seems to be influenced by gender and driven by different aims, both men and women show the innate need to form and maintain interpersonal relationships [7]. Forming and maintaining social bonds have both survival and reproductive benefits [15]. Humans create bonds with other humans in all cultures; as John Donne [16] stated, "No (person) is an island". A lack of supportive relationships triggers emotional distress and has harmful effects on the immune system [17–19].

Relationships satisfy the "need to belong", as it has been called by Baumeister and Leary [20]. Not all relationship bonds, however, satisfy this need—only frequent and pleasant interactions with long-term caring and concern do [20]. According to the authors, "many of the emotional problems for which people seek professional help (anxiety, depression, grief, loneliness, relationship problems, and the like) result from people's failure to meet their belongingness needs".

The communication of emotions plays a fundamental role in forming and maintaining long-term relationships, avoiding potentially dangerous individuals, and moving close to those showing positive emotions toward us or need for help [21]. The most important role among emotions to form intimate relationships seem to be played by sympathy and love [22]. Sympathy, sometimes also called compassion [22], is a care-taking emotion that supports other-oriented, altruistic behavior [23]. Love can be intended as referring to romantic love, familial love, and friendship [24].

These emotions can be conveyed through several nonverbal channels, including face, body, and touch [25]. Some nonverbal channels seem to be more important than others when communicating specific emotional messages [21]. Touch seems to be especially important for fostering intimacy [26] and exhibiting love and sympathy [21]. Moreover, sympathy seems to be accurately communicated by touch only in dyads involving at least one woman, while anger is accurately communicated by touch only in male-only dyads [26]. Opposite-sex dyads, additionally, seem to more accurately recognize touch-expressed love [25].

In addition to gender differences in interpreting touch meaning, we also observe differences in touching behavior: women, compared to men, show more positive attitudes towards and greater willingness to engage in touch with friends and romantic partners [27,28]. However, women are more likely to perceive touch from opposite-sex strangers as unpleasant [27].

In general, the person's attitude toward touching and being touched has been called touch avoidance [27,28]. Touch avoidance is influenced not only by gender but also by attachment processes during infancy and adulthood [29,30]. Attachment theory provides a useful theoretical framework for understanding the importance of touch in development. Bowlby [31] postulated that human touch facilitates the connection between a child and his caregiver, essential for his wellbeing in the early years and beyond. Other studies have demonstrated that during the first year of life, touch influences the child's physical and cognitive development [32] as well as his/her health and sense of safeness [33]. Individual differences in adult attachment security have sometimes been conceptualized in terms of categories, such as secure (individuals not anxious about abandonment nor seeking to avoid others); preoccupied (persons anxious over being abandoned but not avoidant in their behavior), dismissing (people with avoidant behavior without anxiety about being deserted), and fearful (individuals both anxious over abandonment and avoiding closeness) [34].

According to attachment theory, early patterns of tactile behavior and the nature of touch between parents and the child can predict the child's later tendencies to seek or avoid touching people outside the family and attitudes toward touch in adulthood [35]. Indeed, fearful or dismissing individuals avoid and avert touch, unlike secure or preoccupied ones [27,36]. Relationship satisfaction, previous experiences of familial affection, and trust are also positively correlated with mutual touch for romantically involved individuals [37].

Summing up, there is ample evidence of gender differences among women and men on attitudes toward touch, the use of touch for conveying emotions, the importance attributed to relationships, and behavior displayed in social life in general. Since women report higher stress than men, in this study, we want to investigate how gender, attachment, and touch avoidance predict stress responses. Moreover, since the literature is fragmented in describing how different variables leading to stress interact among themselves, the second aim of this study is exploring the network of relationships between gender, attachment, touch avoidance, and stress response.

2. Materials and Methods

2.1. Participants and Procedure

The study was based on a dataset collected for a previous study [38] that involved a total of 335 participants (216 females, 113 males, 6 undisclosed; age = 35.82 ± 14.32, range 16–74) recruited through convenience sampling. We detected no significant gender differences for marital status ($X^2(5) = 1.82$, $p = 0.874$), education $X^2(5) = 8.82$, $p = 0.117$), and occupation ($X^2(16) = 19.63$, $p = 0.237$). Participation was voluntary and anonymous, and participants received no compensation. All tests were completed by pencil-and-paper in a counterbalanced order so as to prevent fatigue and order effects. All missing data (3.5% of responses) were handled through pairwise deletion in all data analyses. This sample size is more than adequate for both multilinear regression (estimated required sample size for 12 predictors, 0.8 power, and moderate effect size ($f^2 = 0.15$) is 127) and network analysis since our network is sparse [39]. R codes and data are available on the repository https://github.com/M-Pass/GenderAndStress.

2.2. Measures

2.2.1. Attachment Style Questionnaire

The attachment style questionnaire (ASQ) [40,41] is a widely used adult attachment measure in both normative and clinical contexts [42]. It comprises 40 items and 5 dimensions. Respondents are asked to indicate their degree of agreement/disagreement with each item on a Likert-type scale ranging from 1 ("strongly disagree") to 6 ("strongly agree"). The ASQ contained five subscales: (a) Confidence (8 items), (b) Discomfort with Closeness (10 items), (c) Relationships as Secondary (8 items), (d) Need for Approval (7 items), and (e) Preoccupation with Relationships (7 items). Discomfort with Closeness refers to Hazan and Shaver's [43] avoidant attachment, whereas Relationships as Secondary is consistent with Bartholomew's [44] concept of dismissing attachment. Need for Approval reflects the respondents' need for acceptance and confirmation from others, referring to Bartholomew's [44] fearful and preoccupied attachment. Lastly, Preoccupation with Relationships involves an anxious and dependent approach to relationships, and Confidence (in Self and Others) reflects a secure attachment orientation. The Italian version of the scale has a Cronbach alpha ranging 0.76–0.84 for the five subscales and 10-week retest reliability ranging 0.67–0.78.

2.2.2. Mesure de Stress Psychologique

The Mesure de Stress Psychologique (MSP) [45,46] is a 49-item self-report questionnaire that measures responses to stress. Each item has a Likert-type response scale ranging from 1 ("not at all") to 4 ("to a great extent"). The final score is computed via software, and the higher the score, the higher the level of stress. The items measure different facets of stress responses, asking the respondent to consider thoughts, somatic symptoms, emotions, and behaviors. The Cronbach alpha for the whole scale is 0.94.

2.2.3. Touch Avoidance Questionnaire

The touch avoidance questionnaire (TAQ) [27,38] assesses attitudes towards touch in different contexts, such as situations involving romantic partners, family members, friends, professional touch, and touch with complete strangers. The TAQ comprises 37 Likert-type items to which participants are asked to respond on a 5-point scale ranging from 1 ("fully disagree") to 5 ("fully agree"). The TAQ subscales are Partner (10 items), Same-sex (6 tems), Opposite-sex (6 items), Family (6 items), and Stranger (3 items). Higher scores indicate higher touch avoidance (i.e., aversion to touch). The Italian version of the scale has an ordinal alpha ranging 0.59–0.92 for the five subscales and 1-month retest reliability ranging 0.67–0.90. Since TAQ Stranger had an ordinal alpha < 0.70, following a reviewer's suggestion, it was removed from the analysis.

2.3. Data Analysis Strategy

Our data analysis strategy encompassed both standard multiple linear regression and techniques originally developed in the network analysis framework. This two-fold data analysis approach serves two separate purposes. First, linear regression—a simple, highly constrained model—can help us ascertain which of the variables being considered has the most direct influence on stress responses (as measured by the MSP), investigating RQ1. Second, network analysis can help us explore the complex web of relationships among the variables in a holistic, data-driven way, investigating RQ2. Since we expect several of the measured constructs to be correlated among themselves and to form a complex causal structure, a technique allowing us to observe all relationships at a glance seemed to us the best fit for this highly explorative study.

3. Results

3.1. Descriptive Statistics and Gender Differences

In Table 1, we report descriptive statistics for the variables considered as well as two-sample t-tests for gender differences. Results show gender differences for viewing relationships as secondary (more common in men) and touch avoidance towards same-sex friends (substantially higher for men). We also observe a gender difference in stress responses bordering significance (t(224,76) = 2.49, p = 0.062, Cohen's d = 0.29).

Table 1. Descriptive statistics for measured variables and *t*-tests for gender differences. ** = significant for $p < 0.01$; *** = significant for $p < 0.001$. All p-values have been adjusted using Benjamini–Hochberg's correction for multiple comparisons.

Variable	Mean and Standard Deviation	Mean and Standard Deviation (Men)	Mean and Standard Deviation (Women)	t-Test for Gender Differences
MSP (Stress responses)	88.86 ± 23.12	84.43 ± 20.39	91.21 ± 24.17	t(224.76) = 2.49, p = 0.062, Cohen's d = 0.29
ASQ1 (Confidence)	32.41 ± 5.15	32.48 ± 4.70	32.39 ± 5.38	t(250) = −0.16, p = 0.939, Cohen's d = 0.02
ASQ2 (Discomfort with Closeness)	35.13 ± 7.94	34.29 ± 6.70	35.54 ± 8.51	t(260.64) = 1.41, p = 0.375, Cohen's d = 0.16
ASQ3 (Relationships as Secondary)	12.89 ± 4.33	14.01 ± 4.66	12.86 ± 4.01	t(186.15) = −3.24, p = 0.010 **, Cohen's d = 0.41
ASQ4 (Preoccupation with Relationships)	20.42 ± 5.81	20.06 ± 5.37	20.59 ± 6.04	t(243.08) = 0.81, p = 0.587, Cohen's d = 0.09
ASQ5 (Need for Approval)	23.19 ± 5.19	22.73 ± 5.03	23.43 ± 5.28	t(226.41) = 1.16, p = 0.436, Cohen's d = 0.13
TAQ—Same Sex	2.07 ± 0.74	2.47 ± 0.81	1.86 ± 0.60	t(117.9) = −7.16, p < 0.001 ***, Cohen's d = 0.91
TAQ—Opposite Sex	2.16 ± 0.74	2.10 ± 0.64	2.18 ± 0.79	t(269.95) = 1.04, p = 0.463, Cohen's d = 0.11
TAQ—Family	2.65 ± 0.96	2.75 ± 0.89	2.60 ± 0.99	t(249.37) = −1.41, p = 0.375, Cohen's d = 0.16
TAQ—Partner	1.94 ± 0.60	1.89 ± 0.53	1.97 ± 0.63	t(257.03) = 1.23, p = 0.436, Cohen's d = 0.14
Age	35.82 ± 14.32	36.40 ± 14.57	35.56 ± 14.23	t(222.81) = −0.50, p = 0.746, Cohen's d = 0.06
Years of scholarization	14.95 ± 3.35	14.59 ± 3.05	15.13 ± 3.50	t(255.75) = 1.44, p = 0.375, Cohen's d = 0.16

MSP = Mesure de Stress Psychologique; ASQ = Attachment Style Questionnaire; TAQ = Touch Avoidance Questionnaire.

3.2. Multiple Linear Regression

As the first part of data analysis, we fitted a multiple linear regression model in which stress responses (as measured by the MSP) are predicted by the four touch avoidance factors of the TAQ (after removal of the "Stranger" subscale), the five factors of the ASQ, gender, age, marital status (coded as "being single"), and years of education. The results are summarized in Table 2. Gender has been coded as 0 = female, 1 = male, and adjusted

R^2 for the whole model is 0.36. The only significant predictors of stress responses seem to be two dimensions of attachment: Confidence and Preoccupation with Relationships, with Discomfort with Closeness bordering on significance (p = 0.062). All associations are in the expected direction: individuals with less confidence, more discomfort with closeness, and more preoccupation exhibited higher stress responses. Additionally, individuals with fewer years of education reported higher stress responses. Importantly, gender was not a significant predictor in the multiple linear regression model, suggesting that the gender-stress response association is spurious.

Table 2. Results of the multiple linear regression model. Df = 226. ** = significant for $p < 0.01$. All p-values have been adjusted using Benjamini–Hochberg's correction for multiple comparisons.

Predictor	Std. β	t	p-Value
(intercept)	0.86	3.26	0.006 **
ASQ1 (Confidence)	−0.24	−3.59	0.006 **
ASQ2 (Discomfort with closeness)	0.16	2.34	0.057
ASQ3 (Relationships as Secondary)	−0.09	−1.56	0.187
ASQ4 (Preoccupation with Relationships)	0.24	3.38	0.006 **
ASQ5 (Need for Approval)	0.10	1.43	0.196
TAQ—Same Sex	−0.10	−1.48	0.196
TAQ—Opposite Sex	0.00	−0.03	0.976
TAQ—Family	0.06	1.10	0.318
TAQ—Partner	0.05	0.93	0.383
Gender	−0.11	−1.76	0.140
Age	−0.12	−1.91	0.121
Marital status (single)	−0.25	−1.89	0.121
Years of education	−0.05	−3.18	0.006 **

MSP = Mesure de Stress Psychologique; ASQ = Attachment Style Questionnaire; TAQ = Touch Avoidance Questionnaire.

3.3. Association Graph

To further explore the relationships among the variables, we computed and plotted a LASSO (least absolute shrinkage and selection operator)-regularized network of partial correlations [39]. Partial correlations are the measure of the residual association between variables X and Y when controlling for all other variables in the network. As such, some variables that appear to be associated when computing 0-order correlations may not be associated when considering partial correlation (as the 0-order correlation is actually spurious). The opposite result is also possible: variables that are associated in the partial correlation network may appear not to be associated when computing 0-order correlations as other variables in the network "mask" their relationship. Partial correlation networks, also called Gaussian graphical models [47] or concentration graphs [48], can be plotted as a weighted network structure in which two variables are connected by an edge if and only if their partial correlation is different from 0 and the edge weight is proportional to the strength of the correlation (ranging from −1 to +1).

To aid interpretability, such a network can be made sparser using LASSO regularization. Partial correlations are rarely exactly zero due to statistical noise and sampling variability. Therefore, plotting the partial correlation network as-is would result in a graph in which all nodes are connected. A widely employed method to solve this problem and avoid over-interpretation of spurious results is regularizing the partial correlation matrix using the LASSO method [49]. LASSO regularization penalizes the likelihood function used for estimating network edges by limiting the sum of (absolute) partial correlations. This results in the shrinkage of all estimated correlations and, most importantly, the lowest correlations shrink to exactly zero. The extent of regularization is controlled by the tuning parameter λ. A lower λ results in less shrinkage, while a higher λ will set more edges to zero and result in a sparse network. The optimal value for λ can be identified by minimizing the EBIC (extended Bayesian information criterion; [50]), a strategy that tends to select the model that best reproduces the underlying true network structure [51]. Additionally, in the reported graph, we removed all edges with a nonsignificant partial correlation.

The resulting graph is shown in Figure 1. From the graph, we can see ASQ1, ASQ2, ASQ4, and ASQ5 remain significantly associated with the MSP even after partializing for all other variables (r = −0.19, p < 0.001; r = 0.20, p = 0.001; r = 0.28, p < 0.001; r = 0.14, p < 0.001).

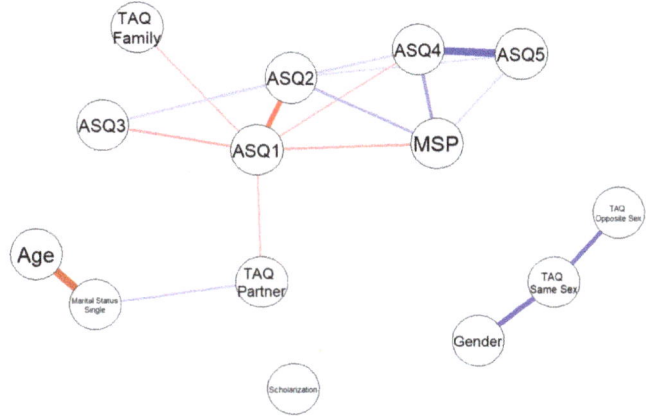

Figure 1. LASSO (least absolute shrinkage and selection operator)-regularized network of partial correlations. Blue lines are positive correlations; red lines are negative correlations. Line width is proportional to partial correlation magnitude.

However, the network also provides us a bird's eye view of all relationships among variables, identifying other important associations. When considering touch avoidance, it is important to note that two factors (touch avoidance towards same-sex friends and opposite-sex friends) are highly related, touch avoidance towards partners is slightly related to touch avoidance towards opposite-sex friends, and touch avoidance towards family members seems to be independent of other measures of touch avoidance. Confidence (ASQ1) is negatively associated to touch avoidance towards family members (r = −0.13, p < 0.001) and romantic partners (r = −0.14, p < 0.001). Additionally, as could be expected, touch avoidance towards partners is associated with being single (r = 0.14, p = 0.001). Notably, while gender is on the periphery of the network, it seems to have a strong relationship with touch avoidance towards same-sex friends (r = 0.053, p < 0.001).

3.4. Causal Discovery

One interesting application of network analysis methods is the use of causal discovery algorithms to infer the directionality of associations.

While finding causal relationships from purely observational, cross-sectional data may seem, at first, impossible, clever use of conditional independence can identify, in some cases, the variable that is the cause and the variable that is the effect [52]. This is the basis of the PC-stable algorithm [53]. The algorithm starts by identifying the skeleton of a graph, i.e., the correlation graph. Then, it identifies triplets of variables X, Y, and Z such that (1) Y is associated with X, (2) Y is associated with Z, (3) X and Z are not associated, and (4) X and Z are associated when partializing for Y. For example, in our data, we have such a situation between the variables Gender, TAQ Same Sex, and TAQ Opposite Sex: Gender and TAQ Opposite Sex are both associated with TAQ Same Sex (r = 0.37 and r = 0.61, respectively) but not with each other (r = 0.05). However, if we condition for TAQ Same Sex, the relationship between gender and TAQ Opposite Sex becomes substantial (r = 0.25). In cases such as this, both edges, X—Y and Z—Y, can be oriented towards Y.

This happens because such a triplet of variables has only four possible configurations: $X \to Y \to Z$, $X \leftarrow Y \leftarrow Z$, $X \leftarrow Y \to Z$, and $X \to Y \leftarrow Z$. However, only the latter would result in conditional dependence between X and Z when conditioning for Y. By directing those edges, the graph implements new constraints that can be used to further direct other edges in the graph. The algorithm thus proceeds iteratively until it directs all edges for which it is possible to infer directionality.

The resulting graph for our data is reported in Figure 2. Note that some of the weaker relationships (e.g., ASQ3–ASQ4) identified in the partial correlation graph are not included in this graph. This is normal and results from the different estimation process used for determining the graph adjacency matrix. Parameters used for the PC-stable algorithm are $\alpha = 0.01$, partial correlations as independence tests, majority rule for checking ambiguous edges, and resolution of conflicts via bidirected edges. This particular setting configuration ensures the algorithm is order-invariant.

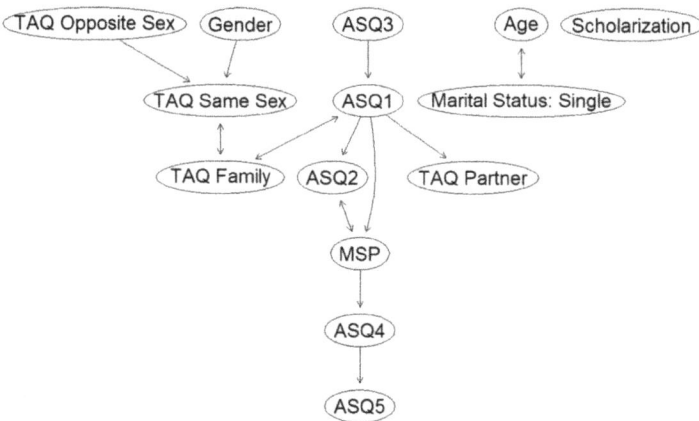

Figure 2. Directed network of the variables' relationships.

Before proceeding with the interpretation of the graph, it should be noted that causal discovery algorithms usually have strict assumptions that are likely to be violated in real-world scenarios. One of the most important ones is that no relevant variables and, especially, no common causes should be omitted from the network. Since this assumption is unlikely to be met, results from the PC-stable algorithm should be interpreted very tentatively. However, the directed graph still offers some suggestions and can be used to inform future research studies.

From the graph, we can see that a direction has been identified for most of the relationships. According to this graph, both gender and touch avoidance of opposite-sex friends exert an influence on same-sex touch avoidance. On the other hand, touch avoidance towards family members is associated both to touch avoidance towards same-sex friends and confidence (ASQ1); however, in both cases, the direction of causality is unclear.

The most interesting region of the graph, however, is the long causal chain involving MSP scores. This chain suggests that viewing relationships as secondary increases confidence, which, in turn, decreases stress responses and touch avoidance towards romantic partners. High levels of stress also heighten preoccupation with relationships, which increases the need for approval. MSP scores are also associated with discomfort with closeness (ASQ2), but it is unclear which variable (if any) is the cause and which is the effect.

4. Discussion

Our results show that some dimensions of attachment, namely, confidence, discomfort with closeness, and preoccupation with relationships, are closely associated with the self-reported intensity of stress responses. According to the causal discovery algorithm, however, it is likely that the level of confidence causes stress responses and that stress responses cause preoccupation with relationships. Attitudes towards touch are not directly related to stress responses, although we observed a substantial gender difference regarding touch with same-sex friends.

Contrary to what would be expected from previous studies [7,8], we surprisingly found age and gender were not significant predictors of stress responses. Indeed, through the network analysis approach, which we used to explore the interrelation of these variables, gender and age were very much on the periphery in the resulting network of variable associations. Interestingly, from our data, it came to light that the variables more strongly related to stress responses all pertain to attachment style. While attitudes towards touch appear to be indirectly associated with stress responses, it is unclear whether one causes the other. Finally, the resulting model highlights additional relationships between variables, suggesting, for example, that attitudes towards touching friends (of either gender) are strongly associated, while attitudes towards touching romantic partners or family members seem to stem from different psychological processes. The strong association found between gender and attitudes towards touching same-sex friends may be related to cultural norms.

This study has important limitations, and its results should be interpreted with caution.

First, the stress response measure—the MSP—conflates the presence of stressors in one's life with the reaction towards these stressors. Indeed, the questionnaire asks respondents how often they experience specific unpleasant responses to stress. Reporting high levels of stress can mean that either the respondent lives in an unusually stressful environment or they are unusually sensitive to daily and ordinary stressful events or both. Replicating the results with a more fine-grained measure of stress would aid the interpretation of how dispositional characteristics interact with life events for determining stress responses. Moreover, a laboratory stress procedure would increase the value of the study, overcoming the limits of self-report instruments.

Second, the methods used in this study—regularized partial correlation networks and causal discovery—are highly suited for exploratory studies but can fail to be replicated in subsequent studies. A replication of these findings, perhaps using a more confirmatory analytical approach, would lend more credibility to our findings.

Third, the study has been conducted in Italy. Since attitudes towards relationships and, especially, social touch differ between cultural contexts [54], future lines of research should focus on testing whether the same causal structure between variables can be observed among the population of other countries.

The causal discovery approach allowed us to find a model that can be used to inform psychological interventions for reducing stress responses, although it bears restating that these results may fail to be replicated and should be interpreted very tentatively. Specifically, the main suggestion emerging from our data is that interventions in clinical settings should focus on improving confidence. One possible way to do so is helping individuals deprived of caring touch during childhood to experience caring and affectionate touch, teaching them to communicate and recognize love and sympathy through touch. Possible approaches for teaching caring touch include compassion-focused therapy [55], in which caring touch is visualized through guided imagery, or functional psychotherapy, in which caring touch is actually employed as a relational tool by a therapist [54]. A second way to improve confidence is helping both men and women strike a balance between their own needs and the needs of their significant others. Mindful self-compassion training, which focuses on the recognition and validation of one's own needs, offers useful tools in this regard [56]. Additionally, our model suggests some important benefits of reducing stress responses, such as improving comfort with closeness and reducing preoccupation with relationships. As a consequence of this result, suggesting client homework such as being massaged by their partner, which could improve their comfort with closeness, could be ineffective if we do not reduce the stress response first. Moreover, intervening on reducing preoccupation with relationships might follow an intervention based on building a sense of confidence and safeness. Gender, instead, appeared to be a mostly inconsequential variable in the network, apart from its strong relationship with same-sex touch avoidance (likely due to social norms). Therefore, gender norms and identity should not be the focus in stress reduction interventions as they are unlikely to play a substantial role.

Lastly, this study also confirms the importance of interventions focused on prevention at a social level to facilitate a secure attachment between parents and children. Since children learn primarily by imitating adults, it would be useful to offer parental training on emotional intelligence and psychological flexibility, with the aim of providing tools for recognizing, validating, and communicating emotions efficiently so as to build pleasant bonds with children in a caring environment [57]. Another important intervention in prevention should consider how to reduce the incidence of postpartum depression. It is well known that depressed mothers report bonding difficulties with their children [58]. Social support and stress interventions during pregnancy have been validated in preventing postpartum depression [59], and efficient interventions have been described to reduce postpartum depression and improve mother–children interactions [60]. However, Italy still lacks a standardized procedure to care for and assess maternal psychological health despite its centrality to parents' and children's wellbeing in the short and long term. In conclusion, our analysis recontextualizes the role of gender in determining responses to stress, suggesting that when we also consider attachment styles and attitudes towards closeness and intimacy, gender appears not to be as central as it would appear at first glance. Interventions in a clinical setting for reducing stress might first consider the client's confidence instead of gender. Moreover, we believe that early prevention could reduce the incidence of stress-related diseases throughout the life-cycle. It should be noted, however, that this study considered an Italian sample and that the relationship between gender, attachment dimensions, attitudes towards touch, and stress responses may differ in other cultural contexts. This is especially true since different genders face different challenges according to societal norms [61], and attitudes towards touch have great variation between cultures [62,63].

5. Limits

The study has some limitations. First of all, the sample is unbalanced (34% males). While the methods used are robust to unbalanced samples, additional data on men could shed more light on the relationship between attachment, stress responses, and touch avoidance.

More importantly, the questionnaire used to assess stress level is ambiguous in what it measures (stressful contexts, stress response attitudes, or both). A more in-depth exploration of stress responses and stressors, based on a sound theoretical framework, could improve our understanding of how gender relates to stress.

Lastly, a more general word of caution is that the methods used (regularized partial correlation networks and causal discovery) to analyze the data are highly suited for exploratory studies but can fail to be replicated in subsequent studies. Additionally, the study was conducted in Italy, so the results cannot be generalized to other countries.

6. Conclusions

This study started from the consideration that women report higher stress than men, even when facing the same stressful events [7,8]. Furthermore, women experience relationships—a major source of both stress and wellbeing—differently from how men experience them, a claim backed by evolutionary psychology [12,13]. Using a highly exploratory design, we investigated in an Italian sample to see if stress responses were predicted by gender, attitudes towards intimacy and closeness (as measured by the attachment Style questionnaire), and attitudes towards interpersonal touch (as measured by the touch avoidance questionnaire). Moreover, we investigated the network of relationships between these variables with the intention of integrating research results that were previously fragmented.

Our results surprisingly recontextualize the role of gender in determining stress responses, as (lack of) confidence, touch avoidance toward family members, and attitudes toward relationships seem to be the main determinants of stress responses.

Overall, our study has important implications in both clinical settings and at a social level. First, clinicians might use these findings and intervene on touch attitudes and lack of confidence to reduce the stress response at its roots. Secondly, our study underlines the importance of prevention at a social level, in particular, psychologically supporting parents from pregnancy throughout the first years of their children's lives in order to build more secure and strong bonds.

Future research should investigate the same topic with different instruments to measure stress response, in particular, employing physiological variables such as heart rate variability or salivary cortisol. Moreover, it would be interesting to evaluate the effectiveness of specific psychological approaches in intervening in the social and relational sphere, comparing their efficacy with those intervening in other spheres such as thoughts, beliefs, and symptoms. These studies could help practitioners improve the efficacy of psychological interventions and reduce their costs and length.

Author Contributions: Conceptualization, M.P., L.C., L.R. and R.P.; methodology, M.P., L.C., L.R. and R.P.; formal analysis, M.P., L.C., L.R. and R.P.; investigation, M.P., L.C., L.R. and R.P.; resources, M.P., L.C., L.R. and R.P.; data curation, M.P., L.C., L.R. and R.P.; writing—original draft preparation, M.P., L.C., L.R. and R.P.; writing—review and editing, M.P., L.C., L.R. and R.P.; visualization, M.P., L.C., L.R. and R.P. All Authors jointly contributed to all phases of the study and of manuscript preparation. All authors have read and agreed to the published version of the manuscript.

Funding: This research received no external funding.

Institutional Review Board Statement: The study was conducted according to the guidelines of the Declaration of Helsinki, and approved by the Ethics Committee of the University of Campania "Luigi Vanvitelli", Department of Psychology (protocol code 4/2019, approved on 29 January 2019).

Informed Consent Statement: Informed consent was obtained from all subjects involved in the study.

Data Availability Statement: Publicly available datasets were analyzed in this study. This data can be found here: https://github.com/M-Pass/GenderAndStress.

Conflicts of Interest: The authors declare no conflict of interest.

References

1. Selye, H. *The Stress of Life*; McGraw Hill: New York, NY, USA, 1956; ISBN 978-0070562127.
2. Anisman, H. The nature of stressors. In *An Introduction to Stress & Health*; SAGE Publications, Inc.: London, UK, 2017; pp. 1–41.
3. Everly, G.S.; Lating, J.M. The anatomy and physiology of the human stress response. In *A Clinical Guide to the Treatment of the Human Stress Response*; Springer: New York, NY, USA, 2019; pp. 19–56.
4. Cohen, S.; Hamrick, N. Stable individual differences in physiological response to stressors: Implications for stress-elicited changes in immune related health. *Brain Behav. Immun.* **2003**, *17*, 407–414. [CrossRef]
5. Charles, S.T.; Piazza, J.R.; Mogle, J.; Sliwinski, M.J.; Almeida, D.M. The wear and tear of daily stressors on mental health. *Psychol. Sci.* **2013**, *24*, 733–741. [CrossRef]
6. Sapolsky, R.M. Individual differences and the stress response. *Semin. Neurosci.* **1994**, *6*, 261–269. [CrossRef]
7. Matud, M.P. Gender differences in stress and coping styles. *Pers. Individ. Dif.* **2004**, *37*, 1401–1415. [CrossRef]
8. Toufexis, D.J.; Myers, K.M.; Davis, M. The effect of gonadal hormones and gender on anxiety and emotional learning. *Horm. Behav.* **2006**, *50*, 539–549. [CrossRef] [PubMed]
9. Holt-Lunstad, J. Why social relationships are important for physical health: A systems approach to understanding and modifying risk and protection. *Annu. Rev. Psychol.* **2018**, *69*, 437–458. [CrossRef] [PubMed]
10. Diener, E.; Oishi, S.; Tay, L. Advances in subjective well-being research. *Nat. Hum. Behav.* **2018**, *2*, 253–260. [CrossRef]
11. Wood, W.; Eagly, A.H. Biosocial construction of sex differences and similarities in behavior. *Adv. Exp. Soc. Psychol.* **2012**, *46*, 55–123. [CrossRef]
12. Symons, D.K.; Buss, D.M. The evolution of desire: Strategies of human mating. *J. Marriage Fam.* **1994**, *56*, 1052. [CrossRef]
13. Meyers-Levy, J.; Loken, B. Revisiting gender differences: What we know and what lies ahead. *J. Consum. Psychol.* **2015**, *25*, 129–149. [CrossRef]

14. Eisenbarth, C. Coping with stress: Gender differences among college students. *Coll. Stud. J.* **2019**, *53*, 151–162.
15. Burkart, J.M. Evolution and consequences of sociality. In *APA Handbook of Comparative Psychology: Basic Concepts, Methods, Neural Substrate, and Behavior*; American Psychological Association: Washington, DC, USA, 2017; pp. 257–271.
16. Donne, J. *Devotions upon Emergent Occasions*; Oxford University Press: Oxford, UK, 1987; ISBN 0375705481.
17. Reed, R.G. Stress and immunological aging. *Curr. Opin. Behav. Sci.* **2019**, *28*, 38–43. [CrossRef] [PubMed]
18. Campagne, D.M. Stress and perceived social isolation (loneliness). *Arch. Gerontol. Geriatr.* **2019**, *82*, 192–199. [CrossRef] [PubMed]
19. Uchino, B.N.; Bowen, K.; de Kent Grey, R.; Mikel, J.; Fisher, E.B. Social support and physical health: Models, mechanisms, and opportunities. In *Principles and Concepts of Behavioral Medicine*; Springer: New York, NY, USA, 2018; pp. 341–372. ISBN 9780387938264.
20. Baumeister, R.F.; Leary, M.R. The need to belong: Desire for interpersonal attachments as a fundamental human motivation. *Psychol. Bull.* **1995**, *117*, 497–529. [CrossRef]
21. App, B.; McIntosh, D.N.; Reed, C.L.; Hertenstein, M.J. Nonverbal channel use in communication of emotion: How may depend on why. *Emotion* **2011**, *11*, 603–617. [CrossRef]
22. Shiota, M.N.; Keltner, D.; John, O.P. Positive emotion dispositions differentially associated with Big Five personality and attachment style. *J. Posit. Psychol.* **2006**, *1*, 61–71. [CrossRef]
23. Goetz, J.L.; Keltner, D.; Simon-Thomas, E. Compassion: An evolutionary analysis and empirical review. *Psychol. Bull.* **2010**, *136*, 351–374. [CrossRef]
24. Fehr, B.; Broughton, R. Gender and personality differences in conceptions of love: An interpersonal theory analysis. *Pers. Relatsh.* **2001**, *8*, 115–136. [CrossRef]
25. Hertenstein, M.J.; Holmes, R.; McCullough, M.; Keltner, D. The communication of emotion via touch. *Emotion* **2009**, *9*, 566–573. [CrossRef]
26. Hertenstein, M.J.; Keltner, D.; App, B.; Bulleit, B.A.; Jaskolka, A.R. Touch communicates distinct emotions. *Emotion* **2006**, *6*, 528–533. [CrossRef]
27. Ozolins, A.; Sandberg, C. Development of a multifactor scale measuring the psychological dimensions of Touch Avoidance. *Int. J. Psychol. A Biopsychosoc. Approach* **2009**, *3*, 33–56.
28. Russo, V.; Ottaviani, C.; Spitoni, G.F. Affective touch: A meta-analysis on sex differences. *Neurosci. Biobehav. Rev.* **2020**, *108*, 445–452. [CrossRef] [PubMed]
29. Ekeberg, D. The Relationship between Interpersonal Touch and Attachment Organization. Master's Thesis, Stockholm University, Stockholm, Sweden, 2016.
30. Johansson, C. Views on and perceptions of experiences of Touch Avoidance: An exploratory study. *Curr. Psychol.* **2013**, *32*, 44–59. [CrossRef]
31. Bowlby, J. *Attachment and loss, Vol. 3: Loss, sadness and depression*; Basic Books: New York, NY, USA, 1980; ISBN 140902024X.
32. Carlson, F.M. Significance of touch in young children's lives. *Young Child.* **2005**, *60*, 79–85.
33. Trevarthen, C.; Aitken, K.J. Infant intersubjectivity: Research, theory, and clinical applications. *J. Child Psychol. Psychiatry* **2001**, *42*, S0021963001006552. [CrossRef]
34. Bartholomew, K.; Horowitz, L.M. Attachment styles among young adults: A test of a four-category model. *J. Pers. Soc. Psychol.* **1991**, *61*, 226–244. [CrossRef]
35. Trotter, P.D.; McGlone, F.; Reniers, R.L.E.P.; Deakin, J.F.W. Construction and validation of the Touch Experiences and Attitudes Questionnaire (TEAQ): A self-report measure to determine attitudes toward and experiences of positive touch. *J. Nonverbal Behav.* **2018**, *42*, 379–416. [CrossRef]
36. Brennan, K.A.; Clark, C.L.; Shaver, P.R. Self-report measurement of adult attachment: An integrative overview. In *Attachment Theory and Close Relationships*; Simpson, J.A., Rholes, S.W., Eds.; Guilford Press: New York, NY, USA, 1998; pp. 46–76. ISBN 1-57230-102-3.
37. Nelson, H.; Geher, G. Mutual grooming in human dyadic relationships: An ethological perspective. *Curr. Psychol.* **2007**, *26*, 121–140. [CrossRef]
38. Casetta, L.; Rizzi, L.; Passarelli, M.; Arcara, G.; Perrella, R. Italian validation of the Touch Avoidance Measure and the Touch Avoidance Questionnaire. *Front. Psychol.* **2020**, *11*, 1673. [CrossRef]
39. Epskamp, S.; Borsboom, D.; Fried, E.I. Estimating psychological networks and their accuracy: A tutorial paper. *Behav. Res. Methods* **2018**. [CrossRef]
40. Feeney, J.A.; Noller, P.; Hanrahan, M. Assessing adult attachment. In *Attachment in Adults: Clinical and Developmental Perspectives*; Sperling, M.B., Berman, W.H., Eds.; Guilford Press: New York, NY, USA, 1994; pp. 128–152. ISBN 0898625475.
41. Fossati, A.; Feeney, J.A.; Donati, D.; Donini, M.; Novella, L.; Bagnato, M.; Acquarini, E.; Maffei, C. On the dimensionality of the attachment style questionnaire in Italian clinical and nonclinical participants. *J. Soc. Pers. Relat.* **2003**, *20*, 55–79. [CrossRef]
42. Fossati, A.; Feeney, J.A.; Donati, D.; Donini, M.; Novella, L.; Bagnato, M.; Carretta, I.; Leonardi, B.; Mirabelli, S.; Maffei, C. Personality disorders and adult attachment dimensions in a mixed psychiatric sample: A multivariate study. *J. Nerv. Ment. Dis.* **2003**, *191*, 30–37. [CrossRef] [PubMed]
43. Hazan, C.; Shaver, P.R. Deeper into attachment theory. *Psychol. Inq.* **1994**, *5*, 68–79. [CrossRef]
44. Bartholomew, K. Avoidance of intimacy: An attachment perspective. *J. Soc. Pers. Relat.* **1990**, *7*, 147–178. [CrossRef]
45. Lemyre, L.; Tessier, R. Mesure de Stress Psychologique (MSP): Se sentir stressé-e. *Can. J. Behav. Sci.* **1988**, *20*, 302–321. [CrossRef]

46. Di Nuovo, S.; Rispoli, L.; Genta, E. Misurare lo stress. In *Il Test MSP e Altri Strumenti per una Valutazione Integrata*; FrancoAngeli: Milan, Italy, 2000; Volume 19.
47. Højsgaard, S.; Edwards, D.; Lauritzen, S.; Højsgaard, S.; Edwards, D.; Lauritzen, S. Gaussian Graphical Models. In *Graphical Models with R*; Springer: New York, NY, USA, 2012.
48. Cox, D.R.; Wermuth, N. A note on the quadratic exponential binary distribution. *Biometrika* **1994**, *81*, 403–408. [CrossRef]
49. Tibshirani, R. Regression Shrinkage and Selection Via the Lasso. *J. R. Stat. Soc. Ser. B* **1996**, *58*, 267–288. [CrossRef]
50. Chen, Z.; Chen, J. Tournament screening cum EBIC for feature selection with high-dimensional feature spaces. *Sci. China Ser. A Math.* **2009**. [CrossRef]
51. Barber, R.F.; Drton, M. High-dimensional Ising model selection with Bayesian information criteria. *Electron. J. Stat.* **2015**, *9*, 567–607. [CrossRef]
52. Hayduk, L.; Cummings, G.; Stratkotter, R.; Nimmo, M.; Grygoryev, K.; Dosman, D.; Gillespie, M.; Pazderka-Robinson, H.; Boadu, K. Pearl's d-separation: One more step into causal thinking. *Struct. Equ. Model. A Multidiscip. J.* **2003**, *10*, 289–311. [CrossRef]
53. Colombo, D.; Maathuis, M.H. Order-independent constraint-based causal structure learning. *J. Mach. Learn. Res.* **2014**, *15*, 3741–3782.
54. Röhricht, F. Body oriented psychotherapy. The state of the art in empirical research and evidence-based practice: A clinical perspective. *Body Mov. Danc. Psychother.* **2009**, *4*, 135–156. [CrossRef]
55. Gilbert, P. An introduction to compassion focused therapy in cognitive behavior therapy. *Int. J. Cogn. Ther.* **2010**, *3*, 97–112. [CrossRef]
56. Germer, C.K.; Neff, K.D. Self-compassion in clinical practice. *J. Clin. Psychol.* **2013**, *69*, 856–867. [CrossRef] [PubMed]
57. Wu, C.-W.; Chen, W.-W.; Jen, C.-H. Emotional intelligence and cognitive flexibility in the relationship between parenting and subjective well-being. *J. Adult Dev.* **2020**. [CrossRef]
58. Hairston, I.S.; Handelzalts, J.E.; Assis, C.; Kovo, M. Postpartum bonding difficulties and adult attachment styles: The mediating role of postpartum depression and child-related PTSD. *Infant Ment. Health J.* **2018**, *39*, 198–208. [CrossRef]
59. Dennis, C.-L.; Dowswell, T. Psychosocial and psychological interventions for preventing postpartum depression. *Cochrane Database Syst. Rev.* **2013**. [CrossRef]
60. Onozawa, K.; Glover, V.; Adams, D.; Modi, N.; Kumar, R.C. Infant massage improves mother–infant interaction for mothers with postnatal depression. *J. Affect. Disord.* **2001**, *63*, 201–207. [CrossRef]
61. Rwafa, U. Culture and religion as sources of gender inequality: Rethinking challenges women face in contemporary Africa. *J. Lit. Stud.* **2016**, *32*, 43–52. [CrossRef]
62. Willis, F.N.; Rawdon, V.A. Gender and national differences in attitudes toward same-gender touch. *Percept. Mot. Skills* **1994**, *78*, 1027–1034. [CrossRef]
63. Burleson, M.H.; Roberts, N.A.; Coon, D.W.; Soto, J.A. Perceived cultural acceptability and comfort with affectionate touch: Differences between Mexican Americans and European Americans. *J. Soc. Pers. Relat.* **2019**, *36*, 1000–1022. [CrossRef]

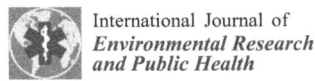

Article

Exploring the Gender Difference and Predictors of Perceived Stress among Students Enrolled in Different Medical Programs: A Cross-Sectional Study

Carmenrita Infortuna [1,†], Francesco Gratteri [1,†], Andrew Benotakeia [2], Sapan Patel [3], Alex Fleischman [3], Maria Rosaria Anna Muscatello [1], Antonio Bruno [1], Rocco Antonio Zoccali [1], Eileen Chusid [3], Zhiyong Han [2] and Fortunato Battaglia [2,*]

1. Department of Biomedical and Dental Sciences and Morphofunctional Imaging, Policlinico Universitario, University of Messina, 98124 Messina, Italy; carmen.infortuna@gmail.com (C.I.); francescogratteri92@icloud.com (F.G.); mmuscatello@unime.it (M.R.A.M.); antonio.bruno@unime.it (A.B.); zoccali@unime.it (R.A.Z.)
2. Department of Medical Sciences and Neurology, Hackensack Meridian School of Medicine at Seton Hall University, Nutley, NJ 07110, USA; andrew.benotakeia@student.shu.edu (A.B.); Zhiyong.han@hackensackmeridian.org (Z.H.)
3. Department of Pre-Clinical Sciences, New York College of Podiatric Medicine, New York, NY 10035, USA; sapanppat@gmail.com (S.P.); afleischman2023@nycpm.edu (A.F.); echusid@nycpm.edu (E.C.)
* Correspondence: fortunato.battaglia@hackensackmeridian.org; Tel.: +1-9737619605
† These authors contributed equally.

Received: 26 July 2020; Accepted: 30 August 2020; Published: 11 September 2020

Abstract: Female medical students seem to experience higher level of perceived stress. Moreover, there is a lack of research examining perceived stress in students enrolled in different medical programs. We analyzed the association between temperament traits, optimism, self-esteem, and perceived stress of students pursuing a Doctor of Medicine (MD) degree and students pursuing a Doctor of Podiatric Medicine (DPM) degree. A cross-sectional study was conducted of two cohorts: allopathic medical students (N = 154) and the podiatric medical students (N = 150). Students anonymously completed the Perceived Stress Scale (PSS-10), Temperament Evaluation of Memphis, Pisa, Paris, and San Diego Auto Questionnaire (TEMPS-A), Rosenberg Self-Esteem Scale, and Life Orientation Test—Revised (LOT-R). We analyzed differences in the two cohort of students and predictors of perceived stress. There were no differences in the overall perception of stress between both cohorts (allopathic medical students: 18.83 ± 0.56; podiatric medical students: 19.3 ± 0.72; $p = 0.4419$). Women reported higher perceived stress in both programs (allopathic medical students: $p = 0.0038$; podiatric medical students: $p = 0.0038$). In both allopathic and podiatric medical students, the cyclothymic temperaments and anxious traits were positive predictors while hyperthymic temperaments and optimism traits were negative predictors of perceived stress. The level of perceived stress experienced by students pursuing different doctoral degrees in healthcare is similar. Regardless of the curriculum differences, female students experience higher perceived stress and there is evidence for similarities in predictors amongst allopathic and podiatric medical students.

Keywords: stress; medical student; temperament; self-esteem; optimism

1. Introduction

In the first two years of graduate medical education, students enrolled in medical schools offering Medical Doctors (MD) degrees and Doctor of Podiatric Medicine (DPM) degrees are introduced to a well-rounded curriculum that encompasses foundational subjects—biochemistry, histology, and immunology—and basic clinical knowledge—pharmacology, radiology, and neuroscience—for preparation for introductory board examinations. Upon a successful completion of board examinations, students continue through a rigorous clinical curriculum spanning two additional years followed by subsequent board examination [1,2]. However, podiatric medical school students hone their specialty with specialized surgical and podiatric medicine courses and clinical hours prior to post-graduate residency [3]. Unlike American medical education, European medical education is a six-year education program. Both American and European medical education require post-medical education residency [4].

Medical students experience a high degree of psychological stress due to frequent examinations, vastness of curriculum, length of training, and high tuition costs [5]. This cumulative effects of stressful experiences in daily life (allostatic loads) may interfere with one's goal [6] and may lead to the development of anxiety and depression over time [7]. Previous studies indicate that female medical students [8–10] experience higher level of distress. Furthermore, the data in the literature are not always consistent [11–14] and the association of gender with the perception of stress in medical student is still be addressed. Thus far, studies comparing the perception of stress in medical students enrolled in different medical programs are lacking. Furthermore, it is yet to be investigated whether the predictors of perceived stress are consistent within the different medical student population.

Stress theory examines the relationship between subjective stress and its contributing factors. In the Transactional Stress model, subjective stress results when threatening and environmental demands of a stressor exceed one's coping resources [15]. Varying perceptions of stress differ from person-to-person even when exposed to the same objective stressor. Thus, several additional factors, such as temperament, optimism, and self-esteem could be associated with the perception of stress and the ability to develop coping strategies. Using the Temperament Evaluation of Memphis, Pisa, Paris, and San Diego-auto-questionnaire short version (TEMPS-A), five temperament dimensions can be described: cyclothymic, depressive, irritable, hyperthymic, and anxious [16]. Previous studies have reported the association between mental distress and specific emotional temperaments and character traits [17–22]. Furthermore, optimism is one's psychological view of life and its possible outcomes. An optimistic perspective drives a friendly, pleasant demeanor and a positive outlook on goals, to which a pessimistic perspective antagonizes [23,24]. Another important factor is self-esteem, that refers to one's view of self-worth. A positive self-esteem increases one's attitude towards themselves, others, and future goals, to which negative self-esteem antagonizes [25]. Low self-esteem increased negative and harmful emotions towards oneself and is associated with stress [26].

To date, there is no study comparing specific mental health factors of graduate medical students enrolled in allopathic and podiatric medical schools. The objectives of this study aimed to compare the following in a cohort of allopathic and podiatric medical school: (i) gender differences in perceived stress levels; (ii) temperament states (cyclothymic, depressive, irritable, hyperthymic, and anxious); (iv) optimism; and (v) self-esteem. The study compared students enrolled in different medical programs (different length of time to graduation, admission requirements, language of study, nationality, medical degree titles, and the influence of culture and tradition) to determine if perceived stress is intrinsic to the medical profession and its education; therefore remaining unaffected by differences in culture or curriculum.

2. Methods

A Cross-sectional study was conducted of two cohorts of students at the allopathic School University of Messina, in Messina, Italy, and the New York College of Podiatric Medicine in New York City, New York. The study was approved by the Institutional Review Boards of the University of Messina and The New York College of Podiatric Medicine and was conducted between June and September 2019. The target population included all students attending preclinical years (the first and second year) at the students of University of Messina Medical School (N = 586) and at the New York College of Podiatric Medicine (N = 190). The study was announced through flyers and social media. Participants were issued an anonymous questionnaire that was returned in a sealed envelope and deposited in a box outside the classroom. The survey contained a statement of consent and the participation was voluntary and anonymous. Population frequencies and variables examined included age, gender, grade point average (GPA), temperament traits, self-esteem, optimism, and perceived stress.

2.1. Measures

Affective temperament traits were evaluated by the Temperament Evaluation of Memphis, Pisa, Paris, and San Diego Auto Questionnaire (TEMPS-A) short version [16]. TEMPS-A questionnaire short version is a 39-question instrument to which participants answer "yes" (1) or "no" (2) [16]. The evaluator scores five subscales (cyclothymic, dysthymic, irritable, hyperthymic, and anxious). The TEMPS-A has good psychometric characteristics [27].

The Rosenberg Self-Esteem Scale quantitatively measures the self-worth of the participant. The Rosenberg Self-Esteem Scale is a 10-question survey which is scored from the extent to which the participants agreed with the questions (from "strongly agree" to "strongly disagree") [28]. Self-esteem correlates to a high final value [28]. The instrument has good psychometric properties [29].

The Life Orientation Test-Revised (LOT-R) quantitatively measures the optimism of the participant. The LOT-R is a 10-questions survey to which four items are not counted. Questions are given a rating from "I agree a lot" to "I disagree a lot" [30]. Psychometric properties were found to be satisfactory [31].

The Perceived Stress Scale—10 (PSS-10) relays quantitative levels of perceived stress [32]. The PSS-10 is a 10-item instrument to which participants rate each listed question about feelings during the past month on a Likert scale (0–4). The PSS-10 has high validity and reliability in medical student population [33].

2.2. Statistical Analysis

Descriptive statistics were conducted to outline medical student's demographic information. Independent t-tests were performed to analyze difference in temperament traits scores, optimism, and self-esteem between allopathic medical students and podiatric medical students. Furthermore, predictors of perceived stress were identified by using two multiple regression models (Model 1: allopathic medical students; Model 2: podiatric medical students). Alpha was set at 0.05 for all statistical tests. Statistical analysis was performed using the Statistical Package for Social Sciences (SPSS, IBM, Armonk, NY, USA) for Windows (version 24.0).

3. Results

The sample consisted of 304 subjects (154 allopathic medical students and 150 podiatric medical students). For allopathic medical students, the mean age of students was 20.88 ± 1.43 with 53.3% of students being female and 46.7% being male. Conversely, podiatric medical students were slightly older (m = 24.17 ± 3.03) with similar gender proportions (60% Female, 40% Male). Lastly, the most significant difference in demographics was ethnicity with allopathic medical students being 100% Caucasian and podiatric medical students being 54% Caucasian, 34% Asian, 10% Hispanic, and 2% African American.

Eight unpaired t-Tests were conducted to compare temperament traits scores, self-esteem, optimism, and perceived stress between both cohorts (Table 1). There was no difference in PSS-10 score between the two cohorts (allopathic medical students: 18.83 ± 0.56; podiatric medical students: 19.3 ± 0.72; p = 0.4419). In both group of students, women displayed higher level of perceived stress (allopathic medical students: t = 1.8; p = 0.041; podiatric medical students: t = 2.23; p = 0.0038). Both allopathic and podiatric medical students showed no significant difference in temperament trait scores: hyperthymic (p = 0.7080), cyclothymic (p = 0.8594), depressive (p = 0.7417), irritable (p = 0.4106), and anxious (p = 0.1422). Similarly, it was found that both allopathic and podiatric medical students showed the same levels of optimism (p = 0.4601) and perceived stress (p = 0.4419). Conversely, podiatric medical students displaced higher self-esteem than allopathic medical students (p = 0.0036).

Table 1. Scores obtained on the five dimensions of the Temperament Evaluation of Memphis, Pisa, Paris, and San Diego questionnaire short version (TEMPS-A), the LOT-R scale, and the Rosenberg Self-Esteem Scale in the allopathic medical students and podiatric medical students. Data are reported as mean ± SE. (**) $p < 0.01$.

Variables	t-Value	p-Value
PSS-10	−0.770	0.4419
Cyclothymic	0.177	0.8594
Depressive	0.330	0.7417
Irritable	0.824	0.4106
Hyperthymic	−0.375	0.7080
Anxious	−1.471	0.1422
LOT-R	0.740	0.4601
Rosenberg scale	−2.933	0.0036 **

Lastly, linear regressions were conducted for both cohorts to determine predictors for perceived stress in allopathic (Model 1) and podiatric (Model 2) medical students. For Model 1, a significant regression equation was found ($F_{(11,156)} = 13.6, p < 0.0001$) with an R^2 of 0.51. The individual predictors were examined further and indicated that cyclothymic ($p < 0.000$) and anxious traits ($p = 0.002$) were positive predictors of perceived stress. On the contrary, hyperthymic trait ($p = 0.001$) and Lot-R scores ($p = 0.002$) were negative predictors (Table 2). Similar results were found when analyzing predictors for perceived stress in podiatric medical students. Model 2 was significant ($F_{(12,149)} = 10.7, p < 0.0001$) with an R^2 of 0.48. Both cyclothymic ($p = 0.03$) and anxious ($p < 0.0001$) temperament scores were positive predictors of perceived. Conversely, both hyperthymic temperament ($p < 0.0001$) and Lot-R scores ($p = 0.045$) were negative predictors of perceived stress for podiatric medical students (Table 3). Self–esteem, depressive, and irritable traits showed no significant predictive value for perceived stress in both models.

Table 2. Multiple regression analysis (Model 1). Predictors of perceived stress in allopathic medical students.

Variables	Unstandardized Coefficients		Standardized Coefficients	t	Sig.	95% Confidence Interval	
	B	Std. Error	Beta			Lower Bound	Upper Bound
(Constant)	13.443	10.306		1.304	0.194	−6.929	33.815
Gender	−0.732	0.914	−0.049	−0.801	0.425	−2.538	1.075
Age	0.296	0.318	0.057	0.933	0.353	−0.332	0.925
Relatives	−0.802	1.063	−0.048	−0.755	0.452	−2.903	1.299
GPA	0.247	0.26	0.057	0.95	0.344	−0.268	0.762
Cyclothymic	0.507	0.101	0.44	5.04	0.000	0.308	0.706
Depressive	0.437	0.219	0.223	1.993	0.058	0.004	0.871
Irritable	−0.47	0.282	−0.259	−1.665	0.098	−1.029	0.088
Hyperthymic	−0.621	0.188	−0.374	−3.294	0.001	−0.993	−0.248
Anxious	1.06	0.339	0.232	3.131	0.002	0.391	1.729
Lot-R	−0.305	0.095	−0.199	−3.221	0.002	−0.492	−0.118
Rosenberg scale	−0.126	0.097	−0.089	−1.292	0.199	−0.318	0.067

Dependent Variables: PSS-10, N = 154.

Table 3. Multiple regression analysis (Model 2). Predictors of perceived stress in podiatric medical students.

Ind. Variables	Unstandardized Coefficients		Standardized Coefficients	t	Sig.	95% Confidence Interval for B	
	B	Std. Error	Beta			Lower Bound	Upper Bound
(Constant)	7.342	5.411		1.357	0.177	−3.359	18.042
Gender	−0.184	0.719	−0.016	−0.256	0.799	−1.606	1.238
Age	−0.08	0.13	−0.039	−0.614	0.54	−0.337	0.177
Ethnicity	−0.24	0.328	−0.047	−0.731	0.466	−0.889	0.409
Relatives	0.863	0.931	0.058	0.927	0.356	−0.978	2.704
GPA	0.24	0.835	0.018	0.287	0.774	−1.411	1.89
Cyclothymic	0.352	0.16	0.154	2.198	0.03	0.035	0.669
Depressive	0.066	0.132	0.032	0.497	0.62	−0.196	0.328
Irritable	−0.047	0.144	−0.021	−0.328	0.743	−0.333	0.238
Hyperthymic	1.445	0.248	0.403	5.829	0.000	0.955	1.936
Anxious	1.379	0.255	0.379	5.409	0.000	0.875	1.883
Lot-R	−0.15	0.078	−0.131	−1.94	0.045	−0.304	0.003
Rosenberg scale	0.112	0.073	0.101	1.524	0.13	−0.033	0.257

Dependent Variables: PSS-10; N = 150.

4. Discussion

Both allopathic and podiatric medical students, despite pursuing different medical programs leading to professions in healthcare with different scopes of practice, showed the same levels of perceived stress. Furthermore, both cohorts of students showed the same predictors of perceived stress. In both cohorts, perceived stress levels were higher in women.

Stress is a determining factor in student well-being and mental health [34]. While the prevalence of stress in allopathic medical students has previously been reported [5,34], investigation of stress in podiatric medical students is lacking. Only one previous study analyzing podiatric medical student well-being revealed a high prevalence of perceived stress, poor sleep quality and excessive daytime sleepiness [14]. Thus, our results fill a gap in the literature and provide, for the first time, comparative data in students pursuing different health professions. Our results confirm previous reports indicating that female medical students show higher level of perceived stress [8,9]. We can only speculate regarding possible determinants. Gender-specific differences in stress reactivity and consequent higher predisposition to depression and anxiety have been previously identified in women [35]. It has been suggested that differences in neuroendocrine and hypothalamic–pituitary–adrenal (HPA) axis reactivity to stress may underlie the higher perception of stress in women [36]. Since both allopathic and podiatric medical students showed similar scores in temperament traits (cyclothymic, depressive, irritable, hyperthymic, and anxious) and similar optimism levels, our results direct towards the importance of stressors rooted in medical school culture rather than difference in burden due to specific curricula (e.g., program duration, scope of practice, type of curriculum, workload, grading system, teaching model, class size, public or private, and administrative resources).

We also found evidence for similar predictors of perceived stress in students enrolled in different programs. For instance, in a clinical population, hyperthymic temperament trait, characterized by having an abnormally positive emotional reaction to daily challenges, has been shown to be a negative predictor for perceived stress [16]. This could possibly be due to fact that individuals with high score in hyperthymic traits are warm, people-seeking, overoptimistic, and exuberant [37]. Thus, those with this trait may be more likely to cope with stressors by sharing problems with family and/or friends, rather than enduring the stressor alone. Additionally, those with higher levels of actionability and responsibility can have a more rapid and effective response to a stress [16]. Optimism has been found to positively influence mental health by counteracting the effect of stress [38] and, in our study, was a negative predictor of perceived stress. Studies by others have indicated that a positive attitude toward life events decreases cortisol secretion and autonomic activation [39–41]. Our result is of pivotal importance since a variety of psychological treatments can boost optimism [42,43], and they could be integrated in psychological support program tailored to reduce abnormal medical student's reaction to the stressful situation.

Cyclothymic temperament trait, characterized by the tendency to quickly change emotional moods, was found to be a positive predictor for increased perceptions of stress. It was shown that cyclothymic temperaments are associated with improper behavioral regulation under naturally occurring stress [17]. The idea that dysregulation of emotions is linked to a greater perception of stress is further supported by the relationship between anxious trait and perceived stress in both groups of students in our study. Anxious temperament trait is characterized by disproportionate levels of nervousness, fear, and apprehension. It was found that those who score high on this trait were unable to discriminate between realistic implications of stressors and exaggerate behavioral responses, and they remain fearful and apathetic towards possible coping strategies [44].

Our results align with proposed theories of stress [15]. This finding also opens an exciting avenue: both hyperthymic temperament and dispositional optimism can predispose students to utilizing more effective coping mechanisms while cyclothymic and anxious traits lead to a self-destructive and harmful coping tactics [45]. Given that our findings show that these effects are largely independent of curricula structure, we believe that they reflect student's response to stressors inherent to medical culture.

This study has some limitation. We employed a cross-sectional study design and, thus, all findings are associations. To determine causality, a prospective study would need to be conducted. Additionally, a study involving a larger number of subjects should be planned to generalize our findings. We should also note the need of a study investigating the impact of different stressors.

5. Conclusions

Our data indicate that, by developing a more optimistic environment in medical schools, allopathic and podiatric medical students would be able to develop a higher resiliency and have less perception of stress. Supporting psychological programs are often utilized for positively impacting psychological and emotional wellbeing of medical students [46]. Because of similarities found between the cohorts in our study, it would be conceivable to design and implement psychological programs incorporating optimism training to be shared by different institutions. Students enrolled in different medical programs could benefit from this experience. In addition, in view of the higher perceived stress level reported in women, future studies are warranted to investigate gender-specific stressors and coping strategies.

Author Contributions: C.I., Investigation, Data Curation, and Software; F.G., Investigation, Data Curation, and Software; A.B. (Andrew Benotakeia), Investigation, Data Curation, Software; and S.P., Investigation, Data Curation, and Software; A.F., Investigation, Data Curation, and Software; M.R.A.M., Conceptualization and Writing—Review and Editing; A.B. (Antonio Bruno), Conceptualization and Writing—Review and Editing; R.A.Z., Conceptualization and Writing—Review and Editing; E.C., Conceptualization and Writing—Review and Editing; Z.H., Conceptualization and Writing—Review and Editing; and F.B., Conceptualization, Supervision, Formal analysis, and Writing—Review and Editing. All authors have read and agreed to the published version of the manuscript.

Funding: This research received no external funding.

Acknowledgments: We thank the students that participated in the study.

Conflicts of Interest: The authors declare no conflict of interest.

References

1. Dezee, K.J.; Artino, A.R.; Elnicki, D.M.; Hemmer, P.A.; Durning, S.J. Medical education in the United States of America. *Med. Teach.* **2012**, *34*, 521–525. [CrossRef] [PubMed]
2. Shannon, S.C.; Teitelbaum, H.S. The status and future of osteopathic medical education in the United States. *Acad. Med.* **2009**, *84*, 707–711. [CrossRef] [PubMed]
3. *New York College of Podiatric Medicine—Academic Catalog*, 2nd ed.; New York College of Podiatric Medicine: New York, NY, USA, 2019.

4. Zavlin, D.; Jubbal, K.T.; Noé, J.G.; Gansbacher, B. A comparison of medical education in Germany and the United States: From applying to medical school to the beginnings of residency. *Ger. Med. Sci.* **2017**, *15*. [CrossRef]
5. Shah, M.; Hasan, S.; Malik, S.; Sreeramareddy, C.T. Perceived stress, sources and severity of stress among medical undergraduates in a Pakistani medical school. *BMC Med. Educ.* **2010**, *10*, 2. [CrossRef] [PubMed]
6. Nechita, F.; Nechita, D.; Pirlog, M.C.; Rogoveanu, I. Stress in medical students. *Rom. J. Morphol. Embryol.* **2014**, *55* (Suppl. 3), 1263–1266.
7. Fava, G.A.; McEwen, B.S.; Guidi, J.; Gostoli, S.; Offidani, E.; Sonino, N. Clinical characterization of allostatic overload. *Psychoneuroendocrinology* **2019**, *108*, 94–101. [CrossRef]
8. Abdulghani, H.M.; AlKanhal, A.A.; Mahmoud, E.S.; Ponnamperuma, G.G.; Alfaris, E.A. Stress and its effects on medical students: A cross-sectional study at a college of medicine in Saudi Arabia. *J. Health Popul. Nutr.* **2011**, *29*, 516–522. [CrossRef]
9. Atkinson, S.R. Elevated psychological distress in undergraduate and graduate entry students entering first year medical school. *PLoS ONE* **2020**, *15*, e0237008. [CrossRef]
10. Al-Sowygh, Z.H. Academic distress, perceived stress and coping strategies among dental students in Saudi Arabia. *Saudi Dent. J.* **2013**, *25*, 97–105. [CrossRef]
11. Casey, D.; Thomas, S.; Hocking, D.R.; Kemp-Casey, A. Graduate-entry medical students: Older and wiser but not less distressed. *Australas. Psychiatry* **2016**, *24*, 88–92. [CrossRef]
12. Quek, T.T.; Tam, W.W.; Tran, B.X.; Zhang, M.; Zhang, Z.; Ho, C.S.; Ho, R.C. The Global Prevalence of Anxiety among Medical Students: A Meta-Analysis. *Int. J. Environ. Res. Public Health* **2019**, *16*, 2735. [CrossRef] [PubMed]
13. Hill, M.R.; Goicochea, S.; Merlo, L.J. In their own words: Stressors facing medical students in the millennial generation. *Med. Educ. Online* **2018**, *23*, 1530558. [CrossRef] [PubMed]
14. Sawah, M.A.; Ruffin, N.; Rimawi, M.; Concerto, C.; Aguglia, E.; Chusid, E.; Infortuna, C.; Battaglia, F. Perceived Stress and Coffee and Energy Drink Consumption Predict Poor Sleep Quality in Podiatric Medical Students A Cross-sectional Study. *J. Am. Podiatr. Med. Assoc.* **2015**, *105*, 429–434. [CrossRef] [PubMed]
15. Lazarus, R.S.; Folkman, S. *Stress, Appraisal, and Coping*; Springer: Berlin/Heidelberg, Germany, 1984.
16. Akiskal, H.S.; Mendlowicz, M.V.; Jean-Louis, G.; Rapaport, M.H.; Kelsoe, J.R.; Gillin, J.C.; Smith, T.L. TEMPS-A: Validation of a short version of a self-rated instrument designed to measure variations in temperament. *J. Affect. Disord.* **2005**, *85*, 45–52. [CrossRef]
17. Goplerud, E.; Depue, R.A. Behavioral response to naturally occurring stress in cyclothymia and dysthymia. *J. Abnorm. Psychol.* **1985**, *94*, 128–139. [CrossRef]
18. Baldessarini, R.J.; Tondo, L.; Pinna, M.; Nunez, N.; Vazquez, G.H. Suicidal risk factors in major affective disorders. *Br. J. Psychiatry* **2019**, 1–6. [CrossRef]
19. Yang, L.; Zhao, Y.; Wang, Y.; Liu, L.; Zhang, X.; Li, B.; Cui, R. The Effects of Psychological Stress on Depression. *Curr. Neuropharmacol.* **2015**, *13*, 494–504. [CrossRef]
20. Jacobshagen, N.; Rigotti, T.; Semmer, N.K.; Mohr, G. Irritation at School: Reasons to Initiate Strain Management Earlier. *Int. J. Stress Manag.* **2009**, *16*, 195–214. [CrossRef]
21. Karam, E.G.; Salamoun, M.M.; Yeretzian, J.S.; Mneimneh, Z.N.; Karam, A.N.; Fayyad, J.; Hantouche, E.; Akiskal, K.; Akiskal, H.S. The role of anxious and hyperthymic temperaments in mental disorders: A national epidemiologic study. *World Psychiatry* **2010**, *9*, 103–110. [CrossRef]
22. Weger, M.; Sandi, C. High anxiety trait: A vulnerable phenotype for stress-induced depression. *Neurosci. Biobehav. Rev.* **2018**, *87*, 27–37. [CrossRef]
23. James, P.; Kim, E.S.; Kubzansky, L.D.; Zevon, E.S.; Trudel-Fitzgerald, C.; Grodstein, F. Optimism and Healthy Aging in Women. *Am. J. Prev. Med.* **2019**, *56*, 116–124. [CrossRef] [PubMed]
24. Oliveira, N.A.; Souza, E.N.; Luchesi, B.M.; Inouye, K.; Pavarini, S.C.I. Stress and optimism of elderlies who are caregivers for elderlies and live with children. *Rev. Bras. Enferm.* **2017**, *70*, 697–703. [CrossRef]
25. Dore, C. Self esteem: Concept analysis. *Rech. Soins Infirm.* **2017**, *129*, 18–26.
26. Kim, D. Relationships between Caregiving Stress, Depression, and Self-Esteem in Family Caregivers of Adults with a Disability. *Occup. Ther. Int.* **2017**, *2017*, 1686143. [CrossRef] [PubMed]
27. Infortuna, C.; Silvestro, S.; Crenshaw, K.; Muscatello, M.R.A.; Bruno, A.; Zoccali, R.A.; Chusid, E.; Intrator, J.; Han, Z.; Battaglia, F. Affective Temperament Traits and Age-Predicted Recreational Cannabis Use in Medical Students: A Cross-Sectional Study. *Int. J. Environ. Res. Public Health* **2020**, *17*, 4836. [CrossRef]

28. Rosenberg, M. Society and the Adolescent Self-Image. *Soc. Forces* **1965**, *44*, 255. [CrossRef]
29. Mark Vermillion, R.A.D. An Examination of the Rosenberg Self-Esteem Scale Using Collegiate Wheelchair Basketball Student Athletes. *Percept. Mot. Ski.* **2007**, *104*, 3. [CrossRef] [PubMed]
30. Scheier, M.F.C.; Charles, S.; Bridges Michael, W. Distinguishing optimism from neuroticism (and trait anxiety, self-mastery, and self-esteem): A reevaluation of the Life Orientation Test. *J. Personal. Soc. Psychol.* **1994**, *67*, 1063–1078. [CrossRef]
31. Glaesmer, H.; Rief, W.; Martin, A.; Mewes, R.; Brähler, E.; Zenger, M.; Hinz, A. Psychometric properties and population-based norms of the Life Orientation Test Revised (LOT-R). *Br. J. Health Psychol.* **2012**, *17*, 432–445. [CrossRef]
32. Cohen, S.; Kamarck, T.; Mermelstein, R.; Mermelstein, T.K. A Global Measure of Perceived Stress. *J. Health Soc. Behav.* **1983**, *24*, 385. [CrossRef]
33. Concerto, C.; Patel, D.; Infortuna, C.; Chusid, E.; Muscatello, M.R.; Bruno, A.; Zoccali, R.; Aguglia, E.; Battaglia, F. Academic stress disrupts cortical plasticity in graduate students. *Stress* **2017**, *20*, 212–216. [CrossRef] [PubMed]
34. Florina Nechita, D.N. Mihail-Cristian Pirlog, Ion Rogoveanu, Stress in medical students. *Rom. J. Morphol. Embryol.* **2011**, *55*, 1263–1266.
35. Kajantie, E.; Phillips, D.I. The effects of sex and hormonal status on the physiological response to acute psychosocial stress. *Psychoneuroendocrinology* **2006**, *31*, 151–178. [CrossRef] [PubMed]
36. Traustadóttir, T.; Bosch, P.R.; Matt, K.S. Gender differences in cardiovascular and hypothalamic-pituitary-adrenal axis responses to psychological stress in healthy older adult men and women. *Stress* **2003**, *6*, 133–140. [CrossRef] [PubMed]
37. Akiskal, H.S.; Placidi, G.F.; Maremmani, I.; Signoretta, S.; Liguori, A.; Gervasi, R.; Mallya, G.; Puzantian, V.R. TEMPS-I: Delineating the most discriminant traits of the cyclothymic, depressive, hyperthymic and irritable temperaments in a nonpatient population. *J. Affect. Disord.* **1998**, *51*, 7–19. [CrossRef]
38. Carver, C.S.; Scheier, M.F.; Fulford, D.; Miller, C.J. Optimism. *Clin. Psychol. Rev.* **2010**, *30*, 879–889. [CrossRef]
39. Russell, G.; Lightman, S. The human stress response. *Nat. Rev. Endocrinol.* **2019**, *15*, 525–534. [CrossRef]
40. Miller, G.E.; Chen, E.; Zhou, E.S. If it goes up, must it come down? Chronic stress and the hypothalamic-pituitary-adrenocortical axis in humans. *Psychol. Bull.* **2007**, *133*, 25–45. [CrossRef]
41. Milam, J.; Slaughter, R.; Verma, G.; McConnell, R. Hair Cortisol, Perceived Stress and Dispositional Optimism: A Pilot Study among Adolescents. *J. Trauma. Stress Disord. Treat.* **2014**, *3*, 1000126.
42. Malouff, J.M.; Schutte, N.S. Can psychological interventions increase optimism? A meta-analysis. *J. Posit. Psychol.* **2017**, *12*, 594–604. [CrossRef]
43. Meevissen, Y.M.; Peters, M.L.; Alberts, H.J. Become more optimistic by imagining a best possible self: Effects of a two week intervention. *J. Behav. Ther. Exp. Psychiatry* **2011**, *42*, 371–378. [CrossRef] [PubMed]
44. Jean, M.; Edwards, K.T. Anxiety, coping and academic performance. *Anxiety Stress Coping* **1992**, *5*, 337–350. [CrossRef]
45. Conway, C.C.; Rutter, L.A.; Brown, T.A. Chronic environmental stress and the temporal course of depression and panic disorder: A trait-state-occasion modeling approach. *J. Abnorm. Psychol.* **2016**, *125*, 10. [CrossRef] [PubMed]
46. Rosenzweig, S.; Reibel, D.K.; Greeson, J.M.; Brainard, G.C.; Hojat, M. Mohammadreza Hojat, Mindfulness-based Stress Reduction Lowers Psychological Distress in Medical Students. *Teach. Learn. Med.* **2003**, *15*, 88. [CrossRef]

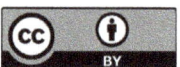

© 2020 by the authors. Licensee MDPI, Basel, Switzerland. This article is an open access article distributed under the terms and conditions of the Creative Commons Attribution (CC BY) license (http://creativecommons.org/licenses/by/4.0/).

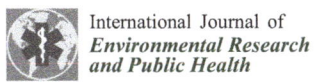

Review

Psychological Impact of Pro-Anorexia and Pro-Eating Disorder Websites on Adolescent Females: A Systematic Review

Carmela Mento [1,*], Maria Catena Silvestri [2], Maria Rosaria Anna Muscatello [1], Amelia Rizzo [2], Laura Celebre [1], Martina Praticò [1], Rocco Antonio Zoccali [1] and Antonio Bruno [1]

1. Department of Biomedical, Dental Sciences and Morphofunctional Imaging, University of Messina, Psychiatric Unit Policlinico "G. Martino" Hospital, 98124 Messina, Italy; mmuscatello@unime.it (M.R.A.M.); lallacelebre@gmail.com (L.C.); martinapratico@hotmail.com (M.P.); rocco.zoccali@unime.it (R.A.Z.); antonio.bruno@unime.it (A.B.)
2. Psychiatric Unit, Policlinico Hospital "G. Martino", 98124 Messina, Italy; mariacate@libero.it (M.C.S.); amrizzo@unime.it (A.R.)
* Correspondence: cmento@unime.it

Abstract: (1) Background: Teenagers (in particular, females) suffering from eating disorders report being not satisfied with their physical aspect and they often perceive their body image in a wrong way; they report an excessive use of websites, defined as PRO-ANA and PRO-MIA, that promote an ideal of thinness, providing advice and suggestions about how to obtain super slim bodies. (2) Aim: The aim of this review is to explore the psychological impact of pro-ana and pro-mia websites on female teenagers. (3) Methods: We have carried out a systematic review of the literature on PubMed. The search terms that have been used are: "*Pro*" AND "*Ana*" OR "*Blogging*" AND "*Mia*". Initially, 161 publications were identified, but in total, in compliance with inclusion and exclusion criteria, 12 studies have been analyzed. (4) Results: The recent scientific literature has identified a growing number of Pro Ana and Pro Mia blogs which play an important role in the etiology of anorexia and bulimia, above all in female teenagers. The feelings of discomfort and dissatisfaction with their physical aspect, therefore, reduce their self-esteem. (5) Conclusion: These websites encourage anorexic and bulimic behaviors, in particular in female teenagers. Attention to healthy eating guidelines and policies during adolescence, focused on correcting eating behavioral aspects, is very important to prevent severe forms of psychopathology with more vulnerability in the perception of body image, social desirability, and negative emotional feedback.

Keywords: eating abnormal behavior; pro-ana and pro-mia websites; female adolescents

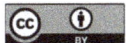

1. Introduction

Eating disorders are multifactorial disorders, affecting about 0.3% of female teenagers; they have a prevalence included between 1.2% and 4.2%. In particular, anorexia nervosa arises during adolescence, and it can be devastating, potentially included suicidal risk [1–3]. A common trait among young women with eating disorders is low self-esteem, with a tendency towards depressed moods. Many factors seem to influence the development and preservation of these disorders among female teenagers. The scientific panorama shows how teenagers with eating disorders have a distorted body image, an wrong perception of their image, and therefore, are more dissatisfied with their physical aspect, in comparison to celebrities. Body image can generate feelings of satisfaction or dissatisfaction and this can cause the individual to make radical choices when treating his/her body [4,5]. In this context, there are a variety of pro-eating disorder communities (websites), and teenagers use social media to talk about their physical aspect, their activities, and to exchange advice about weight loss; this condition supports anorexia nervosa, as the problem of weight loss becomes relevant for their lives and the solution to their health problems. In fact, according to the scientific literature, all members of these communities have reported high levels of eating disorders [6].

Pro-ana and pro-mia websites are virtual spaces, in which teenagers can exchange ideas about their body image and physical aspect. An uncontrolled use of these websites is common practice among teenagers, in particular among young women, and is a factor related to eating disorders. In this regard, some years ago, several authors started to include addiction to the Internet and eating disorders among problematic behaviors in adolescents. Frequent use of social networks and the possibility to follow celebrities (e.g., influencers, models, actors, and actresses) influence perception of the self and of one's own physical and psychological way of being. This happens when there is a social meeting that can influence the user's (teenager) mood. This desire to look like celebrities on social networks can promote the insurgence and/or preservation of eating disorders such as anorexia and bulimia. The influence of social media is growing among female teenagers with advice and tips to lose weight and showing images of thin bodies.

In line with different studies, looking at images of underweight celebrities is associated to an ideal body image and aspiration to lose weight and these conditions can promote eating disorders [7,8].

Pro-ana and pro-mia websites offer feedback on people's physical aspect: teenagers receive comments on their aspect and advice on how to lose weight [9–17]. These forums are private and the topic being dealt with is the philosophy of absolute thinness [18–20]. In recent years, a study by Almenara and colleagues [21] demonstrated that looking for sensations and disinhibition online were both associated with a higher risk of exposure to ana–mia websites for teenage women and young adults. According to Borzekowski et al. (2010), most websites (58%) contain images of celebrities with ultra slim bodies and promote an anorexic lifestyle, and teenagers visiting pro-ana websites seem to have higher levels of body dissatisfaction and eating disorders [10].

Bates (2015) examined the metaphors used in a pro-ana website to talk about oneself. The author has applied the Metaphor Identification Procedure to 757 text profiles and has identified four key metaphorical constructions in self-description by pro-ana members: self as space, self as weight, and improving the self and social self. Bert and colleagues (2016) found 341 pro-ana accounts on Twitter; for each account, the authors analyzed the number of followers, users' biographical information, and have studied the most used hashtags. These accounts were very popular, having 23.609 followers; users were mainly young women (97.9 percent) and teenagers. This study demonstrated that the most used hashtags were: "thinspiration", "proana", "thin15", "'ana tips". These accounts contain dangerous information about body image, eating habits, and physical aspect. Bragazzi et el. (2019) studied 402 websites and demonstrated that the media tend to spread images of models who are abnormally thin.

In a previous study, Çelik and colleagues (2015) found a positive correlation between problematic use of the Internet and approach to food, and the problematic use of the Internet predicted these approaches [22]. The dimension of the effect in relation to the negative impact of pro-ED websites is related to eating pathology. Several authors have counted a large number of websites promoting dysfunctional eating behaviors such as anorexia and bulimia [23–26].

In light of the collected data in the scientific literature, the aim of this report is to explore the psychological impact of pro-ana and pro-mia websites on female teenagers.

2. Materials and Methods

Data for this systematic review have been collected in compliance with the reporting elements used for systematic reviews and meta-analysis [27]. PRISMA consists of a checklist aimed at making preparation and reporting of review/meta-analysis studies easier, by identifying, selecting, and critically assessing analyzed research and analyzing data from the studies included in the review.

2.1. Criteria for Eligibility

The articles have been included in the review according to the following inclusion criteria: English language, publication in peer reviewed journals, quantitative information on language processing in movement disorders, and year of publication from 2015—2020. Articles have been excluded according to title, abstract, or complete text for the processes linked to the psychological impact of pro-ana and pro-mia websites on adolescents and to irrelevance to the topic being dealt with. Further exclusion criteria were review articles, editorial comments, and case reports/series. Moreover, it was arbitrarily decided to start our research in 2015 to provide a more recent outlook on the psychological impact of pro-ana and pro-mia websites among teenagers.

2.2. Research Strategy

This systematic review has been carried out according to systematic review guidelines [27]. The PubMed database has been searched from 1 January 2015 to 1 January 2020, using 4 key terms related to this topic ("Pro" AND "Ana" OR "Blogging" AND "Mia"). The electronic research strategy used for PubMed is described in Table 1. The articles have been selected according to title and abstract; the entire article has been read if the title/abstract was related to the specific issue of the psychological impact of pro-ana and pro-mia websites on female teenagers and if the article potentially met inclusion criteria. Moreover, references to the selected articles have been examined in order to identify further studies which could meet the inclusion criteria.

Table 1. List of search terms entered into PubMed.

Number	Search Term
1	Pro (all fields)
2	Ana (all fields)
3	Blogging (all fields)
4	Mia (all fields)
5	1 AND 2
6	OR 3 AND 4
7	English (Language)
8	2015/01/01 to 2020/01/01 (publication date)

2.3. Search Strategy and Study Selection

Overall, bibliographical research has been carried out in the PubMed database, with final research updated to January 2020. Initial research used key terms "Pro" AND "Ana" OR "Blogging" AND "Mia". The key terms used are related to processes connected to the psychological impact of pro-ana and pro-mia websites or blogs.

Figure 1 sums up the flow chart of the articles selected for review. Research in the PubMed database provided a total of 161 quotations; no additional studies meeting the inclusion criteria were identified when checking the reference list of the selected documents.

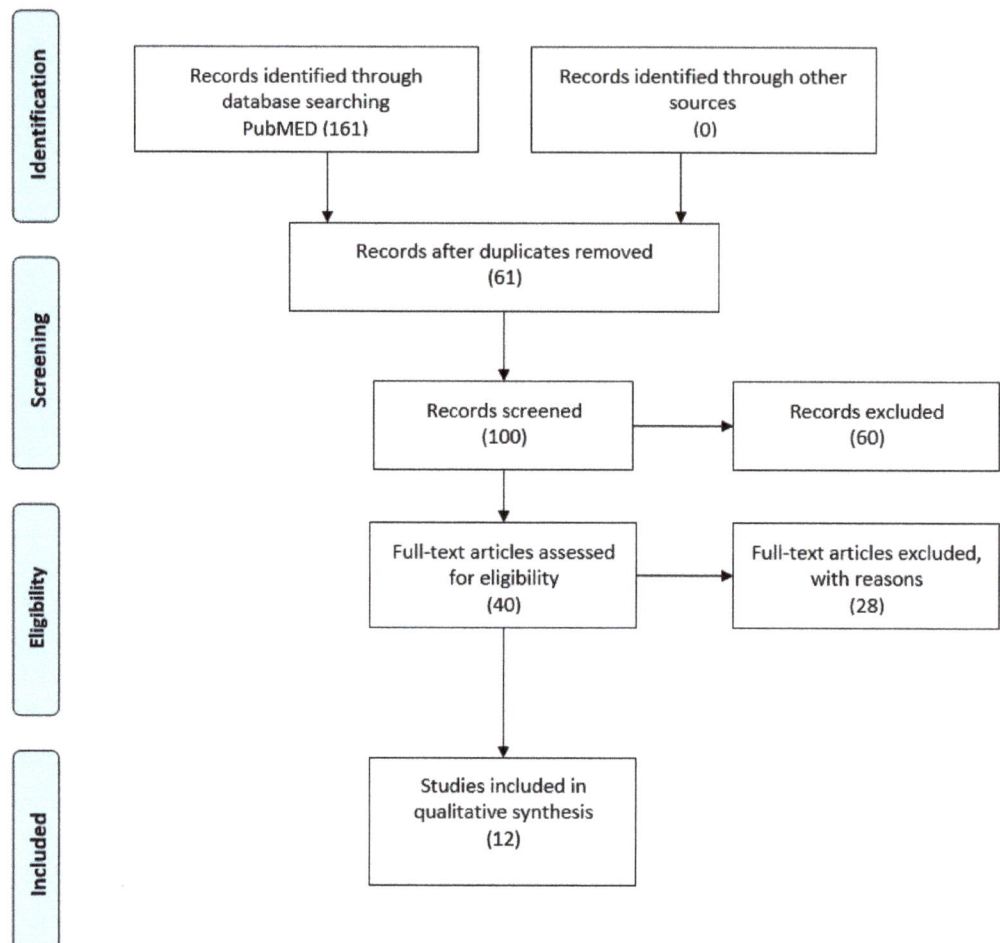

Figure 1. PRISMA (2009) flow diagram.

After checking duplicate copies, 61 records have been examined. Among these, 28 studies have been excluded, based on inclusion and exclusion criteria. After the screening, a total of 12 studies, having checked the processes connected to the psychological impact of pro-ana and pro-mia websites on female teenagers, have met the inclusion criteria and have been included in the systematic review (Table 2).

Table 2. Characteristics of the studies included in the review.

Author	Aim	Sample	Type of Measure	Findings
Almenara et al., (2016)	This study explored the individual differences associated with adolescents' exposure to "ana-mia" websites.	N = 18,709 girls, aged 11–16, 50%	-Exposure to "ana-mia" websites -Daily use of the Internet -Digital skills -Online disinhibition -Sensation seeking -Socioeconomic status of the household.	The results of this study showed that sensation seeking and online disinhibition were both associated with an increased risk of exposure to "ana-mia" websites in girls as well as in boys, although some gender differences were apparent. In girls, but not in boys, the older the child and higher the socioeconomic status, higher the chance of being exposed to "ana-mia" websites.
Bates (2015)	This study examined the metaphors the members of a pro-ana group invoked in their personal profiles on a popular social networking site, to talk about the self.	757 text profiles.	-The Metaphor Identification Procedure to 757 text profiles.	This study identified four key metaphorical constructions in pro-ana members' self-descriptions: self as space, self as weight, perfecting the self, and the social self. These four main metaphors represented discourse strategies, both to create a collective pro-ana identity and to enact an individual identity as pro-ana.
Bert et al., (2016)	The aim of this study is to investigate the presence, popularity, and content of the "proana" accounts on Twitter.	341 accounts.	-Investigated the most used hashtags and the main contents of these profiles. -Twitter search. -For the statistical analysis of the retrieved data, used Stata MP11.	The authors found high number and popularity of Twitter proanorexia groups. These accounts contain dangerous information, especially considering the young age of the users.
Bragazzi et al., (2019)	The aim of the current investigation was to systematically perform a reliability and content analysis of Italian language anorexia nervosa-related websites.	402 unique website.	- Health on the Net Foundation Code of Conduct Standards (HonCode®) certification mark.	This study showed that the quality of Italian language anorexia nervosa-related websites was rather moderate-poor, being generally inconsistent with the principles of the HonCode® certification mark.
Çelik et al., (2015)	The aim of this study was to investigate the relationship between problematic internet use and eating attitudes in a group of university students.	students.	-The Problematic Internet Use Scale -Eating Attitudes Test -Personal Data Form.	The research findings showed a significant positive correlation between problematic internet use and eating disorders, the problematic internet use is a predictor of eating disorders.
Chang & Bazarova (2016)	The aim of this study was to explore online negative enabling support dynamics in pro-anorexic websites through the language analysis of initiating disclosure and response sequences.	Analyzing 22,811 messages from 5590 conversations from the Pro-Ana Nation online discussion board forum.	- Linguistic Analysis.	The findings showed that initiating disclosures containing stigma-related emotion words, anorexia-specific content, and sociorelational content are typically met with negatively valenced responses from other members of the pro-anorexic community.
Gale et al., (2015)	The present study aimed to explore the underlying functions and processes related to the access and continued use of pro-ED websites within a clinical eating disorder population using a qualitative research design.	Seven adult women in treatment for an eating disorder who had disclosed current or historic use of pro-ED websites. Interviewees ranged in age from 20 to 40 years.	-Face-to-face semistructured interviews.	This study showed that Pro eating disorder websites maintaining eating disordered behaviour. This websites appeared to offer a sense of support for adolescents with eating disorder.
Hernández-Morante et al., (2015)	The objective of this study was to determine both general and information quality of eating disorder websites, including obesity websites.	50 websites.	- Three key terms (obesity, anorexia and bulimia) were entered into the Google®search engine. Websites were assessed using two tests (HonCode®certification and Bermudez-Tamayo et al. test) to analyze overall quality, and a third test (DISCERN test) to analyze specifically information quality.	This study determinated that the pro eating web sites influenced the eating disorders, including obesity.

Table 2. *Cont.*

Author	Aim	Sample	Type of Measure	Findings
Hilton (2018)	The aim of this study was to studied the Qualitative Exploration of the Role of Pro-anorexia Websites in User's Disordered Eating.	151 members of pro-ana website.	- The analysis revealed five main themes: eating disorders are mental illnesses and websites do not cause mental illness, pro-ana websites and eating disorders.	This research revealed the role of pro anorexia websisites in eating disorders.
Tan et al., (2016)	The aim of this study was to assess a group of patients with eating disorders in Singapore who presented for treatment.	56 participants.	-Eating Disorder Examination Questionnaire 6.0 (EDE-Q 6.0) -Eating Attitudes Test26 (EAT-26) -Clinical Impairment Questionnaire 3.0 (CIA 3.0).	This study looked at the Internet and smartphone app usage patterns of participants who presented with an eating disorder in Singapore, and whether it corresponded to severity of illness. Overall, any smartphone application usage was associated with younger age and greater eating disorder psychopathology and psychosocial impairment.
Yom-Tov et al., (2016)	The aim of the current study is to explore the characteristics of people who participate in different pro-anorexia web communities and the differences between them.	Posts from the discussion board of the myproana.com website (A total of 57,911 post).	Identified users who used the terms in the 5 categories above. For those users, the most popular terms were categorized as follows: Myproana: users who queried for the myproana.com website. Tumblr: users who queried for the social network tumblr, Manorexia: users who queried for the term "manorexia", meaning anorexia in males, Thinspiration, Yahoo Answers: visitors to the popular Yahoo Answers website.	Members of the main pro-ana website investigated appear to be depressed, with high rates of self-harm and suicide attempts, users are significantly more interested in treatment, have wishes of procreation and reported the highest goal weights among the investigated sites.
Yom-Tov et al., (2018)	The objective of this randomized controlled trial (RCT) was to examine if online advertisements (ads) can change online search behaviors of users who are looking for online pro-ana content.	10 different Bing Ads system.	-Using the Bing Ads system.	Exposure to the pro eating disorder websites, was associated an increased of eating disorders.

The selected studies have demonstrated the relationship between pro-anorexia and pro-bulimia websites/forums and eating behaviors; a variety of studies have dealt with this topic, in particular research on the relation between pro-ana and pro-mia websites and the desire to lose weight.

This review has examined the psychological impact of pro-ana and pro-mia websites on female teenagers. Articles have been selected according to title and abstract; the entire article has been read if the title/abstract was related to the specific issue of the psychological impact of pro-ana and pro-mia websites on female teenagers in relation to eating disorders; and if the article potentially met the inclusion criteria. Details are reported in Tables 1 and 2. Additionally, references to the selected articles have been examined in order to identify further studies which could meet inclusion criteria (Table 3).

Table 3. Prisma checklist.

Section/Topic	#	Checklist Item	Reported on Page #
Title			
Title	1	Psychological Impact of Pro-Anorexia and Pro-Eating Disorders Websites on Adolescent Females: A systematic review	1
Abstract			
Structured summary	2	The studies present in the literature showed that the websites defined as pro-ana and pro-mia supported eating disorders in female adolescents, because these websites promote an ideal of an ultra-thin body. The aim of this review is to explore the psychological risk of pro-ana and pro-mia websites in female adolescents. We carried out a systematic review of the literature on PubMed. We used the terms "Pro" AND "Ana" OR "Blogging" AND "Mia". In the initial search, we identified 161 publications, and a total of 12 studies were selected according to inclusion criteria. The inclusion criteria were: English language, publication in peer reviewed journals, quantitative information on pro-ana and pro-mia websites among adolescents, in particular female adolescents, review articles, editorial comments, and case reports, and year of publication at least after 2015. We arbitrarily decided to start our research from 2015 to give a more recent view of the psychological impact of pro-ana and pro-mia websites on female adolescence findings. The PubMed database was searched from January 1 2015 to January 1 2020. According to the scientific literature, female adolescents were dissatisfied with their physical appearance, and the inappropriate use of the Internet increased the risk of eating disorders. It is very important to pay attention to this condition, to promote healthy eating habits, and to prevent the risk of eating disorders.	1, 3, 4, 5
Introduction			
Rationale	3	Many factors seem to influence the development and preservation of eating disorders among female teenagers. The scientific panorama shows how teenagers with eating disorders have a distorted body image, an inaccurate perception of their image, and therefore, are more dissatisfied with their physical aspect, in comparison to celebrities. There are a variety of pro-eating disorders communities (websites), and teenagers use social media to talk about their physical aspect, their activities, and to exchange advice about weight loss; this condition supports anorexia nervosa, as the problem of weight loss becomes relevant for their lives and the solution to their health problems. In fact, according to the scientific literature, all members of these communities have reported high levels of eating disorders.	2
Objectives	4	The aim of this work is to explore the psychological risk of pro-ana and pro-mia websites among female adolescents.	2
Methods			
Protocol and registration	5	We used these search terms: "Pro" AND "Ana" OR "Blogging" AND "Mia". In the initial search, we identified 161 publications, but after, according to inclusion and exclusion criteria, we analyzed 12 studies.	
Eligibility criteria	6	We used these eligibility criteria: English language, publication in peer reviewed journals, studies about pro-ana and pro-mia websites and female adolescents, and year of publication at least after 2015. Articles were excluded by title, abstract, or full text for irrelevance to the topic. Exclusion criteria were: review articles, editorial comments, and case reports/series. We arbitrarily decided to start our research from 2015 to give a more recent view of "the psychological impact of pro-ana and pro-mia websites on female adolescents".	3
Information sources	7	This systematic review was conducted according to Systematic Reviews guidelines. The PubMed database was searched from January 1 2015 to January 1 2020, using 4 key terms related to this topic ("Pro" AND "Ana" OR "Blogging" AND "Mia").	3, 4
Search	8	Articles have been selected by title and abstract; the entire article was read if the title/abstract was related to the specific issue of the psychological impact of pro-ana and pro-mia on adolescents, and if the article potentially met the inclusion criteria. References of the selected articles were also examined in order to identify additional studies meeting the inclusion criteria.	4

Table 3. *Cont.*

Section/Topic	#	Checklist Item	Reported on Page #
Study selection	9	A comprehensive literature search was conducted in PubMed database, with the final search updated on January 2020. The initial search conducted used the keywords "Pro" AND "Ana" OR "Blogging" AND "Mia". We used key terms related to the processes connected to the psychological impact of pro-ana and pro-mia websites or blogging.	4
Data collection process	10	The search of the PubMed database provided a total of 161 citations; no additional studies meeting the inclusion criteria were identified by checking the reference list of the selected papers. After adjusting for duplicates, 61 records were screened. Of these, 28 studies were excluded according to the inclusion and exclusion criteria. After the screening, a total of 12 studies assessing the processes connected to the psychological impact of pro-ana and pro-mia websites on adolescents met the inclusion criteria and were included in the systematic review.	4
Data items	11	Not specified.	
Risk of bias in individual studies	12	Across the included studies in this review, a potential database bias should be considered. Only articles written in English language were used, which might have compromised access to articles published in other languages.	5
Summary measures	13	"ana-mia" websites	1,2,3
Synthesis of results	14	Most of the research analyzed was focused on the negative impact of these websites on female adolescents, such as anorexia and bulimia.	5
Section/topic	#	Checklist item	Reported on page #
Risk of bias across studies	15	In all studies included in this review, a potential bias of the database should be considered. Only articles in English have been used, which could have compromised access to articles published in other languages.	5
Additional analyses	16	Not specified.	
Results			
Study selection	17	Record articles we identified on PubMed (n = 161); records identified through other sources (n = 0); records after duplicates removed (n = 61); records screened (n = 100); records excluded (n = 60); full-text articles assessed for eligibility (n = 40); full-text articles excluded; with reasons (n = 28); studies included in qualitative synthesis (n = 12).	Figure 1
Study characteristics	18	Almenara et al. (2016) studied the individual differences in adolescents on "ana-mia" websites, in a sample of N = 18,709 girls, aged 11–16, 50%. The authors used these types of measure: exposure to "ana-mia" websites; daily use of the Internet; digital skills; online disinhibition; sensation seeking; socioeconomic status of the household. Bates (2015) studied the metaphors used in pro-ana. Bert et al. (2016) studied 341 accounts on these websites. Bragazzi et al. (2019) studied the language in anorexia nervosa-related websites. Çelik et al. (2015) investigated the relationship between problematic internet use and eating attitudes in a group of university students. Chang and Bazarova (2016) explored online negative enabling support dynamics in pro-anorexic websites through language. Gale et al. (2015) studied pro-ED websites. Hernández-Morante et al. (2015): the objective of this study was to determine both general and information quality of eating disorder websites, including obesity websites; they studied 50 websites and three key terms (obesity, anorexia, and bulimia) were entered into the Google®search engine. Hilton (2018) studied the Qualitative Exploration of the Role of Pro-anorexia Websites in User's Disordered Eating. Yom-Tov et al. (2016, 2018) explored the characteristics of adolescents who participate in different pro-anorexia web communities.	Table 2
Risk of bias within studies	19	In all studies in this review, a potential bias of the database should be considered. Only articles in English, which could have compromised access to articles published in other languages	

Table 3. Cont.

Section/Topic	#	Checklist Item	Reported on Page #
Results of individual studies	20	The recent scientific literature has identified a growing number of pro-ana and pro-mia blogs which play an important role in the etiology of anorexia and bulimia, above all in female teenagers. The feeling of discomfort and dissatisfaction with their physical aspect therefore reduces their self-esteem	5
Synthesis of results	21	Most analyzed research has focused on the negative influence of websites in female adolescents with eating disorders such as anorexia and bulimia. These websites have seemed to offer a sense of support to teenagers vulnerable to eating disorders. These studies have explored adolescent exposure to these websites, personal profiles related to access to social network, as well as pro-ana accounts on Twitter [18,21,26,28]. Other more social, aspects, linked to communication and language, have been explored in a recent study on language and information used on this website [29–31]. The relationship between a problematic use and abuse of the Internet and eating behaviors in adolescence has been investigated, as well as negative online support in the case of pro-anorexia websites [11,14,22]. Psychological aspects are generally explored as a potential risk of eating disorders to exacerbate or preserve symptoms of users' eating disorders in a sample population [17,32]. Another study has explored the physical and mental state of people participating in pro-anorexia web communities [33]. In particular, Almenara and colleagues (2016) have demonstrated that looking for sensations and disinhibition online were both associated with a higher risk of exposure to ana–mia websites, in male and female teenagers, although some gender differences were evident. In girls, but not among boys, the older the teenager was and the higher her socioeconomic status was, the higher the chances were of being exposed to "ana-mia" websites. Bates (2015) identified four key metaphorical constructions in self-description by pro-ana members: self as space, self as weight, and improving the self and social self. These four main metaphors represented speech strategies, both in order to create a collective pro-ana identity and to enact an individual identity as pro-ana. Bert et al. (2016) highlighted a high number and popularity pro-anorexia groups on Twitter. These accounts contain dangerous information, especially considering the users' young age. The investigation by Bragazzi et al. (2019) aimed at carrying out a systematic analysis of the reliability and content of websites related to anorexia nervosa in the Italian language. Çelik et al. (2015) have shown a significant positive correlation between a problematic use of the Internet and eating disorders. A problematic use of the Internet is a predictor of eating disorders. Chang and Bazarova (2016) have demonstrated that publications containing emotional words linked to stigma, the specific content of anorexia, and very correlational content generally trigger negative feedback from other members of the pro-anorexia community. Gale et al. (2015) demonstrated that pro-eating disorder websites lead to preserving the behavior of the eating disorder. These websites seemed to offer a sense of support to teenagers with eating disorders. Hernández-Morante et al. (2015) have stated that pro-eating disorder websites influence eating behavior, including obesity. Hilton (2018) has shed light on the role of pro-anorexia websites in eating disorders. Tan et al. (2016) have examined models of Internet and smartphone apps for individuals showing eating disorders in Singapore and checked if they corresponded to the severity of the disease. Overall, any use of applications for smartphones was associated with a younger age and a higher psychopathology of eating disorders and psychosocial deficit. Yom-Tov et al. (2016) have explored the characteristics of people participating in different pro-anorexia web communities and the differences among them, and have shown that the women members of the main pro-ana website investigated seem to be depressed.	8
Risk of bias across studies	22	In all studies included in this review, a potential bias of the database should be considered. Only articles in English have been used, which could have compromised access to articles published in other languages	5
Additional analysis	23	Not specified.	
Discussion			
Summary of evidence	24	Several authors have identified many bloggers focused on pro-anorexic lifestyles and diets, giving advice and tips on how to lose weight (such as laxatives, purging in the shower, excessive exercise, calorie restriction, slimming pills, limitations in eating habits), extreme thinness, negative messages about food, and information about body image. Researchers have studied other aspects that can promote eating habits such as competition among members of these blogs to lose weight and be thin. Members of these communities would like to use their body image as inspiration models.	8

Table 3. *Cont.*

Section/Topic	#	Checklist Item	Reported on Page #
Limitations	25	The limitations of this study were the poor empirical studies to describe these phenomena.	8
Conclusions	26	As highlighted in the scientific literature, pro-ana and pro-mia websites promote a negative approach to food in a vulnerable population, such as in teenagers, and these conditions can encourage insurgence of eating disorders. Explaining this phenomenon connected to the use of forums and websites among female teenagers is fundamental because anorexia and bulimia are very serious and dangerous diseases, with higher incidence in the period of teenage development. However, it is very important to identify online content and raise awareness on the level of danger on these websites and on maladaptive eating approaches among young people. Different studies have found out that a negative image of the self can limit quality of life and pro-anorexia and pro-bulimia websites do not cause eating disorders but can encourage them. As far as the research topic is concerned, it is necessary to implement actions of promotion of guidelines and policies for healthy eating habits in the target population. Some aspects are relevant to improve the impact of research on prevention in the teenage population because at the moment, there are not many empirical studies in the literature explaining it. The need to prematurely recognize maladaptive signs, words, beliefs, and approaches in a teenager can indicate healthy eating guidelines and policies with specific programs of school education, even for teachers and parents. These healthy eating contexts can raise awareness on problematic eating behaviors and identify cases needing counselling and treatment or, in the most serious cases, hospitalization, therefore reducing the potential for a wide range of teenagers being trapped in the net. Further research to understand the correlation between personality profile and the impact of exposure to "Ana-mia" websites on prevention of mental health in teenagers is recommended. The issue is relevant in young populations to prevent the risk of suicide and psychopathological and mental problems in adulthood.	7,8
Funding			
Funding	27	The author(s) received no financial support for the research, authorship, and/or publication of this article	8

From: (Mother et al., 2009) related to Prisma Checklist form [27].

2.4. Bias Risk among Studies

In all studies included in this review, a potential bias of the database should be considered. Only articles in English have been used, which could have compromised access to articles published in other languages.

3. Results

Most analyzed research has focused on the negative influence of websites in female teenagers with eating disorders such as anorexia and bulimia. These websites have seemed to offer a sense of support to teenagers vulnerable to eating disorders. These studies have explored teenagers' exposure to these websites, personal profiles related to popular access to social network, as well as pro-ana accounts on Twitter [18,21,26,28]. Other more social aspects, linked to communication and language, have been explored in a recent study on language and information used on this website [29–31]. The relationship between a problematic use and abuse of the Internet and eating behaviors in adolescents has been investigated, as well as negative online support in the case of pro-anorexia websites [11,14,22]. Psychological aspects are generally explored as a potential risk of eating disorders to exacerbate symptoms of users' websites eating disorders in a sample population [17,32]. Another study has explored the physical and mental state of people participating in pro-anorexia web communities [33]. In particular, Almenara and colleagues (2016) have demonstrated that looking for sensations and disinhibition online were both associated with a higher risk of exposure to ana–mia websites, in male and female teenagers, although some gender differences were evident. In girls, but not among boys, the older the teenager was and the higher her socioeconomic status was, the higher the chances were of being exposed to "ana-mia" websites. Bates (2015) has identified four key metaphorical constructions in self-description by pro-ana members: self as space, self as weight, and improving the self and social self. These four main metaphors represented speech strategies, both in order to create a collective pro-ana identity and to enact an individual identity as pro-ana. Bert et al. (2016) have highlighted a high number and popularity pro-anorexia groups on Twitter. These accounts contain dangerous information, especially considering the users' young ages. The investigation by Bragazzi et al. (2019) aimed at carrying out a systematic analysis of the reliability and content of websites related to anorexia nervosa in the Italian language. Çelik et al. (2015) have shown a significant positive correlation between a problematic use of the Internet and eating disorders. A problematic use of the Internet is a predictor of eating disorders. Chang and Bazarova (2016) demonstrated that publications containing emotional words linked to stigma, the specific content of anorexia, and very correlational content generally trigger negative feedback from other members of the pro-anorexia community. Gale et al. (2015) have demonstrated that pro-eating disorder websites lead to preserving the behavior of the eating disorder. These websites seemed to offer a sense of support to teenagers with eating disorders. Hernández-Morante et al. (2015) have stated that pro-eating disorder websites influence eating behaviors, including obesity. Hilton (2018) has shed light on the role of pro-anorexia websites in eating disorders. Tan et al. (2016) have examined models of Internet and smartphone apps, for individuals showing eating disorders. Overall, any use of applications for smartphones was associated with a younger age and a higher psychopathology of eating disorders and psychosocial deficit. Yom-Tov et al. (2016) have explored the characteristics of people participating in different pro-anorexia web communities and the differences among them, and have shown that the women members of the main pro-ana website investigated seem to be depressed.

4. Discussion

According to the scientific literature, eating disorders are a serious psychiatric disease, with a mortality rate going from 5 to 6 percent, higher than all other mental disorders. In particular, anorexia is difficult to treat and, in the cyberspace, there is a phenomenon of pro-eating disorder websites, in particular pro-anorexia, that means there are many websites supporting anorexia—pro-ana and pro-mia. The aim of these websites is to promote an anorexic lifestyle. These websites can encourage unhealthy habits and in particular, can promote eating disorders [28,29]. Most analyzed research is focused on the social effects of pro-ana and pro-mia websites, and different authors have demonstrated that they most frequently are visited by the young female population [34–36]. However, some recent research suggests that pro-ana and pro-mia websites can encourage negative eating behaviors, such as promoting a pro-anorexic approach, through suggestions and tips to lose weight. The literature mainly examines the social influence of the media and has shown that these websites and blogs show ideal images of absolute thinness [37–39].

Several authors have identified many bloggers focused on pro-anorexic lifestyles and diets, giving advice and tips on how to lose weight (such as laxatives, purging in the shower, excessive exercise, calorie restriction, slimming pills, limitations in eating habits), extreme thinness, negative messages about food, and information about body image. Researchers have studied other aspects that can promote eating habits such as competition among members of these blogs to lose weight and be thin. Members of these communities would like to use their body image as inspiration models, for example, in the website's gallery. This is in line with anti-recovery, because these blogs, communities, and/or websites reject recovery and medical treatment for eating disorders. Another form of resistance involved in these websites is disagreement with psychiatric and psychological treatment [30–35].

Most users of these websites are teenagers and have a complex psychological relationship with food—maybe they use it as a reward, a punishment, or they even feel guilty for eating some specific hypercaloric foods. According to the epidemiology of eating disorders, many accounts on pro-ana and pro-mia websites are managed by girls and in 58% of cases, websites contain images intended to encourage weight loss. Young women are particularly vulnerable to this kind of website, are attracted to them, and in fact, the most common people visiting pro-eating disorder websites are 13-, 15-, and 17-year-olds [10].

An important cognitive aspect found is connected to recursive thought. Sharing emotions is maladaptive when users, instead of reconsidering a negative event, continue to brood over it. Thinking continuously makes a negative event more enjoyable and prevents individuals from distraction, therefore intensifying stress, anxiety, shame, and other negative emotions associated with that event [40]. Brooding over a negative event and its meaning, without cognitively reconsidering that event, has proven to intensify negative emotions, making users even more depressed, anxious, and angry in comparison to the initial self-revelation. In these websites, users through pro-ana and pro-mia forums always brood over the same topic. Results have shown that mainly young women feel uncomfortable and often dissatisfied with their body image, and have consequently reduced their self-esteem and have difficulty in relational and social activities [41,42].

However, there is a limited number of empirical studies in the literature on the topic that have investigated the risks associated with the development of eating psychopathology in adolescents. The existing literature on pro-eating disorder websites has not focused on clinical and psychopathological behaviors that can lead also to a serious risk of suicide in young populations. It is very important to focus on the risk of using websites and forums encouraging maladaptive eating habits, especially in vulnerable teenagers with problems linked to food. Higher behavioral risks in the use of eating disorder websites show a higher tendency to isolation, negative emotions, and maladaptive eating habits, which can be predictors of eating disorders or can exacerbate subclinical pictures in vulnerable subjects.

The paper highlights the importance of a study focused on the psychological impact of pro-ana and pro-mia websites in female teenagers with vulnerabilities in eating habits. The psychological impact of images, texts, words, and of a maladaptive eating approach for an ultra-slim body is an extremely complex process, and is dangerous for teenagers' body image. There are many psychological and identity development factors, as well as socio-cognitive skills and aspects of social desirability that are involved.

Our results suggest the importance of paying attention to psychoeducation among teenagers about eating disorders, food nutritional principles, and provide correct information on factors preparing, precipitating, or preserving the insurgence of eating disorders. This plays an important role in order to improve quality in their life and to reduce the risk of eating disorders.

5. Limitations

A limitation of the present study is the scarce literature on this topic. There are few empirical studies that explain the psychological motivation that attracts adolescents to eating websites.

6. Conclusions

As highlighted in the scientific literature, pro-ana and pro-mia websites promote a negative approach to food in a vulnerable population, such as in adolescents, and these conditions can encourage the insurgence of eating disorders.

Explaining this phenomenon connected to the use of forums and websites among female teenagers is fundamental because anorexia and bulimia are very serious and dangerous diseases, with higher incidence in the period of teenage development. However, it is very important to identify online contents and raise awareness on the level of danger of these websites and on maladaptive eating approaches among young people. Different studies have found out that a negative self-image can limit quality of life and pro-anorexia and pro-bulimia websites do not cause eating disorders but can encourage them. As far as the research topic is concerned, it is necessary to implement actions of promotion of guidelines and policies for healthy eating habits in the target population. Some aspects are relevant to improve the impact of research on prevention in the teenage population because at the moment, there are not many empirical studies in the literature explaining it.

The need to prematurely recognize maladaptive signs, words, beliefs, and approaches in adolescents for healthy eating guidelines and policies with specific programs of school education, even for teachers and parents. These healthy eating contexts can raise awareness on problematic eating behaviors and identify cases needing counselling and treatment or, in the most serious cases, hospitalization, therefore reducing the potential for a wide range of teenagers being trapped in the net. Further research to understand the correlation between personality profile and the impact of exposure to "Ana-mia" websites on the prevention of mental health issues in teenagers is recommended. The issue is relevant in young populations to prevent the risk of suicide and psychopathological and mental problems in adulthood.

Author Contributions: Conceptualization C.M. and M.R.A.M.; methodology M.C.S. and A.B.; da-ta curation, C.M., M.C.S. and M.P.; writing—original draft preparation C.M., M.R.A.M., R.A.Z.; writing—review and editing C.M., A.R., L.C., M.C.S. All authors have read and agreed to the published version of the manuscript.

Funding: The authors received no financial support for the research, authorship, and/or publication of this article.

Institutional Review Board Statement: Not applicable.

Informed Consent Statement: Not applicable.

Data Availability Statement: The study did not report any data.

Conflicts of Interest: The authors declared no potential conflict of interest with respect to the research, authorship, and/or publication of this article.

References

1. Yom-Tov, E.; Fernandez-Luque, L.; Weber, I.; Crain, S.P.; Lewis, S. Pro-Anorexia and Pro-Recovery Photo Sharing: A Tale of Two Warring Tribes. *J. Med. Internet Res.* **2012**, *14*, e151. [CrossRef] [PubMed]
2. Arts, H.; Lemetyinen, H.; Edge, D. Readability and quality of online eating disorder information—Are they sufficient? A systematic review evaluating websites on anorexia nervosa using DISCERN and Flesch Readability. *Int. J. Eat. Disord.* **2020**, *53*, 128–132. [CrossRef]
3. Delforterie, M.J.; Larsen, J.K.; Bardone-Cone, A.M.; Scholte, R.H.J. Effects of Viewing a Pro-Ana Website: An Experimental Study on Body Satisfaction, Affect, and Appearance Self-Efficacy. *Eat. Disord.* **2014**, *22*, 321–336. [CrossRef]
4. Fichter, M.M.; Quadflieg, N.; Nisslmüller, K.; Lindner, S.; Osen, B.; Huber, T.; Wünsch-Leiteritz, W. Does internet-based prevention reduce the risk of relapse for anorexia nervosa? *Behav. Res. Ther.* **2012**, *50*, 180–190. [CrossRef]
5. Gumz, A.; Uhlenbusch, N.; Weigel, A.; Wegscheider, K.; Romer, G.; Löwe, B. Decreasing the duration of untreated illness for individuals with anorexia nervosa: Study protocol of the evaluation of a systemic public health intervention at community level. *BMC Psychiatry* **2014**, *14*, 300. [CrossRef]
6. Hötzel, K.; Von Brachel, R.; Schmidt, U.; Rieger, E.; Kosfelder, J.; Hechler, T.; Schulte, D.; Vocks, S. An internet-based program to enhance motivation to change in females with symptoms of an eating disorder: A randomized controlled trial. *Psychol. Med.* **2014**, *44*, 1947–1963. [CrossRef] [PubMed]
7. Schlegl, S.; Bürger, C.; Schmidt, L.; Herbst, N.; Voderholzer, U. The Potential of Technology-Based Psychological Interventions for Anorexia and Bulimia Nervosa: A Systematic Review and Recommendations for Future Research. *J. Med. Internet Res.* **2015**, *17*, e85. [CrossRef]
8. Varns, J.A.; Fish, A.F.; Eagon, J.C. Conceptualization of body image in the bariatric surgery patient. *Appl. Nurs. Res.* **2018**, *41*, 52–58. [CrossRef]
9. Yom-Tov, E.; Boyd, D.M. On the link between media coverage of anorexia and pro-anorexic practices on the web. *Int. J. Eat. Disord.* **2014**, *47*, 196–202. [CrossRef] [PubMed]
10. Borzekowski, D.L.G.; Schenk, S.; Wilson, J.L.; Peebles, R. e-Ana and e-Mia: A Content Analysis of Pro–Eating Disorder Web Sites. *Am. J. Public Health* **2010**, *100*, 1526–1534. [CrossRef]
11. Chang, P.F.; Bazarova, N.N. Managing Stigma: Disclosure-Response Communication Patterns in Pro-Anorexic Websites. *Health Commun.* **2016**, *31*, 1–13. [CrossRef]
12. Hamilton, K.; Waller, G. Media Influences on Body Size Estimation in Anorexia and Bulimia. *Br. J. Psychiatry* **1999**, *162*, 837–840. [CrossRef] [PubMed]
13. Field, A.E.; Cheung, L.; Wolf, A.M.; Herzog, D.B.; Gortmaker, S.L.; Colditz, G.A. Exposure to the Mass Media and Weight Concerns Among Girls. *Pediatrics* **1999**, *103*, e36. [CrossRef] [PubMed]

14. Gale, L.; Channon, S.; Larner, M.; James, D. Experiences of using pro-eating disorder websites: A qualitative study with service users in NHS eating disorder services. *Eat. Weight. Disord.-Stud. Anorex. Bulim. Obes.* **2016**, *21*, 427–434. [CrossRef] [PubMed]
15. Oksanen, A.; García, D.; Räsänen, P. Proanorexia Communities on Social Media. *Pediatrics* **2016**, *137*, e20153372. [CrossRef]
16. Rodgers, R.F.; Skowron, S.; Chabrol, H. Disordered eating and group membership among members of a pro-anorexic online community. *Eur. Eating Disorders Rev.* **2012**, *20*, 9–12. [CrossRef]
17. Rouleau, C.R.; Von Ranson, K.M. Potential risks of pro-eating disorder websites. *Clin. Psychol. Rev.* **2011**, *31*, 525–531. [CrossRef]
18. Bates, C.F. "I am a waste of breath, of space, of time" metaphors of self in a pro-anorexia group. *Qual. Health Res.* **2015**, *25*, 189–204. [CrossRef]
19. Boepple, L.; Thompson, J.K. A content analytic comparison of fitspiration and thinspiration websites. *Int. J. Eat. Disord.* **2016**, *49*, 98–101. [CrossRef]
20. Knapton, O. Pro-anorexia: Extensions of ingrained concepts. *Discourse Soc.* **2013**, *24*, 461–477. [CrossRef]
21. Almenara, C.A.; Machackova, H.; Smahel, D. Individual Differences Associated with Exposure to "Ana-Mia" Websites: An Examination of Adolescents from 25 European Countries. *Cyberpsychol. Behav. Soc. Netw.* **2016**, *19*, 475–480. [CrossRef]
22. Çelik, Ç.B.; Odacı, H.; Bayraktar, N. Is problematic internet use an indicator of eating disorders among Turkish university students? *Eat. Weight. Disord.-Stud. Anorex. Bulim. Obes.* **2015**, *20*, 167–172. [CrossRef]
23. Rodgers, R.F.; Lowy, A.S.; Halperin, D.M.; Franko, D.L. A Meta-Analysis Examining the Influence of Pro-Eating Disorder Websites on Body Image and Eating Pathology. *Eur. Eat. Disord. Rev.* **2016**, *24*, 3–8. [CrossRef]
24. Daga, G.A.; Gramaglia, C.; Pierò, A.; Fassino, S. Eating disorders and the Internet: Cure and curse. *Eat. Weight. Disord. Stud. Anorex. Bulim. Obes.* **2006**, *11*, e68–e71. [CrossRef]
25. Bardone-Cone, A.M.; Cass, K.M. What does viewing a pro-anorexia website do? An experimental examination of website exposure and moderating effects. *Int. J. Eat. Disord.* **2007**, *40*, 537–548. [CrossRef] [PubMed]
26. Yom-Tov, E.; Brunstein-Klomek, A.; Mandel, O.; Hadas, A.; Fennig, S.; Milton, A.; Chen, T.; Rodgers, R. Inducing Behavioral Change in Seekers of Pro-Anorexia Content Using Internet Advertisements: Randomized Controlled Trial. *JMIR Ment. Health* **2018**, *5*, e6. [CrossRef]
27. Moher, D.; Liberati, A.; Tetzlaff, J.; Altman, D.G. Preferred reporting items for systematic reviews and meta-analyses: The PRISMA statement (Chinese edition). *J. Chin. Integr. Med.* **2009**, *7*, 889–896. [CrossRef]
28. Bert, F.; Gualano, M.R.; Camussi, E.; Siliquini, R. Risks and Threats of Social Media Websites: Twitter and the Proana Movement. *Cyberpsychol. Behav. Soc. Netw.* **2016**, *19*, 233–238. [CrossRef] [PubMed]
29. Bragazzi, N.L.; Prasso Gre, T.S.; Zerbetto, R.; Del Puente, G.A. Reliability and content analysis of Italian language anorexia nervosa-related websites. *Risk Manag. Healthc. Policy* **2019**, *12*, 145. [CrossRef]
30. Hernández-Morante, J.J.; Jiménez-Rodríguez, D.; Cañavate, R.; Conesa-Fuentes, M.D.C. Analysis of Information Content and General Quality of Obesity and Eating Disorders Websites. *Nutr. Hosp.* **2015**, *32*, 606–615.
31. Hilton, C.E. "It's the Symptom of the Problem, Not the Problem itself": A Qualitative Exploration of the Role of Pro-anorexia Websites in Users' Disordered Eating. *Issues Ment. Health Nurs.* **2018**, *39*, 865–875. [CrossRef]
32. Tan, T.; Kuek, A.; Goh, S.E.; Lee, E.L.; Kwok, V. Internet and smartphone application usage in eating disorders: A descriptive study in Singapore. *Asian J. Psychiatry* **2016**, *19*, 50–55. [CrossRef]
33. Yom-Tov, E.; Brunstein-Klomek, A.; Hadas, A.; Tamir, O.; Fennig, S. Differences in physical status, mental state and online behavior of people in pro-anorexia web communities. *Eat. Behav.* **2016**, *22*, 109–112. [CrossRef]
34. Kelly, T.M.; Yang, W.; Chen, C.-S.; Reynolds, K.D.; He, J. Global burden of obesity in 2005 and projections to 2030. *Int. J. Obes.* **2008**, *32*, 1431–1437. [CrossRef]
35. Hinojo-Lucena, F.-J.; Aznar-Díaz, I.; Cáceres-Reche, M.-P.; Trujillo-Torres, J.-M.; Romero-Rodríguez, J.-M. Problematic Internet Use as a Predictor of Eating Disorders in Students: A Systematic Review and Meta-Analysis Study. *Nutrients* **2019**, *11*, 2151. [CrossRef] [PubMed]
36. Jett, S.; Laporte, D.J.; Wanchisn, J. Impact of exposure to pro-eating disorder websites on eating behaviour in college women. *Eur. Eat. Disord. Rev.* **2010**, *18*, 410–416. [CrossRef] [PubMed]
37. Boero, N.; Pascoe, C. Pro-anorexia Communities and Online Interaction: Bringing the Pro-ana Body Online. *Body Soc.* **2012**, *18*, 27–57. [CrossRef]
38. Day, K.; Keys, T. Anorexia/bulimia as resistance and conformity in pro-Ana and pro-Mia virtual conversations. In *Critical Feminist Approaches to Eating Disorders*; Moulding, N., Ed.; Routledge: London, UK, 2012; pp. 109–118.
39. Lladó, G.; González-Soltero, R.; De Valderrama, M.J.B.F. Anorexia y bulimia nerviosas: Difusión virtual de la enfermedad como estilo de vida. *Nutr. Hosp.* **2017**, *34*, 693. [CrossRef] [PubMed]
40. Rimé, B.; Finkenauer, C.; Luminet, O.; Zech, E.; Philippot, P. Social Sharing of Emotion: New Evidence and New Questions. *Eur. Rev. Soc. Psychol.* **1998**, *9*, 145–189. [CrossRef]
41. De Vries, D.; Peter, J.; De Graaf, H.; Nikken, P. Adolescents' Social Network Site Use, Peer Appearance-Related Feedback, and Body Dissatisfaction: Testing a Mediation Model. *J. Youth Adolesc.* **2016**, *45*, 211–224. [CrossRef]
42. Pavan, C.; Marini, M.; De Antoni, E.; Scarpa, C.; Brambullo, T.; Bassetto, F.; Mazzotta, A.; Vindigni, V. Psychological and Psychiatric Traits in Post-bariatric Patients Asking for Body-Contouring Surgery. *Aesthetic Plast. Surg.* **2017**, *41*, 90–97. [CrossRef] [PubMed]

MDPI
St. Alban-Anlage 66
4052 Basel
Switzerland
Tel. +41 61 683 77 34
Fax +41 61 302 89 18
www.mdpi.com

International Journal of Environmental Research and Public Health Editorial Office
E-mail: ijerph@mdpi.com
www.mdpi.com/journal/ijerph

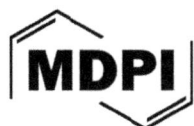

www.ingramcontent.com/pod-product-compliance
Lightning Source LLC
LaVergne TN
LVHW070603100526
838202LV00012B/553